THE PALEO CHEF

THE PALEO CHEF

Quick, Flavourful Paleo
Meals for Eating Well

PETE EVANS

Photography by
Mark Roper

MACMILLAN

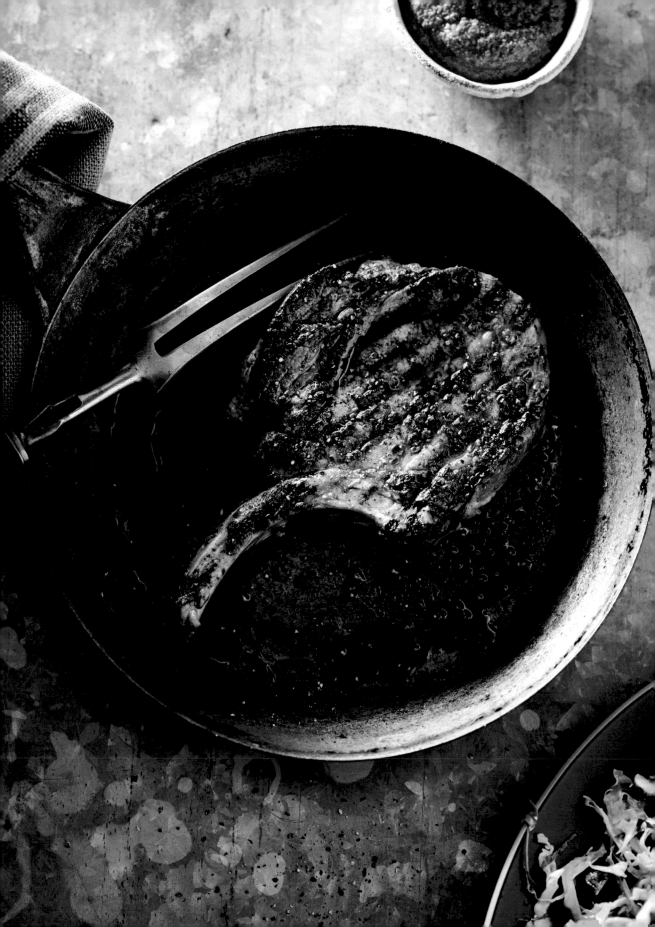

CONTENTS

foreword

Change is afoot in the world of the professional kitchen. Every day more and more people are realizing that the quality of what we put in our bodies directly impacts our sense of balance, our health, our happiness, and our overall well-being. A few simple changes to how we eat, a little consideration for our ingredients, and we see great changes in how we feel. A considerate approach to how we eat is helping countless people reclaim their health. It's worked for me — I've recovered from a so-called 'incurable' autoimmune disease and I attribute the lion's share of my recovery to the foods that I eat.

No chef I know is nearly as passionate as Pete Evans when it comes to eating for health and happiness and making sure not to forget the pleasure. This important book closes the door, once and for all, on the stigma of healthy food not being delicious food. In Pete's kitchen, eating for nourishment is pleasurable and passionate and full of love. As we've strayed farther from the foods we ate in the recent past, we've begun to pay the price with longer, sicker lives. And while food may be but a piece in the puzzle of our growing health crisis, it's one that we can take control over. Pete's craveable recipes like Mum's Burgers or Roasted Winter Vegetables are decadent, indulgent, and supremely good for us. He brilliantly creates food that is both familiar and innovative, all the while up-ending the conventional notion of what it means to eat for wellness.

—

Much of the diet and health trends in food over the past thirty years — focusing on calorie restriction and synthetic low-fat foods, demonizing saturated fats (which the mainstream is starting to realize are not at the root of our food-related health problems), and promoting a food pyramid that upheld inflammatory foods like whole grains as the cornerstone of our diets — have done more harm to our well-being than good. Through this, the Paleo movement has quietly grown. As it's grown, more and more people, myself included, have seen amazing changes in their bodies and huge progress in how they feel, overcoming seemingly insurmountable obstacles. Pete's book illustrates how Paleo is a personal path with guidelines, but without rules, and with a celebration of food, flavour, and wellness in every bite.

Seamus Mullen
Chef and Proprietor, Tertulia and El Colmado, New York City

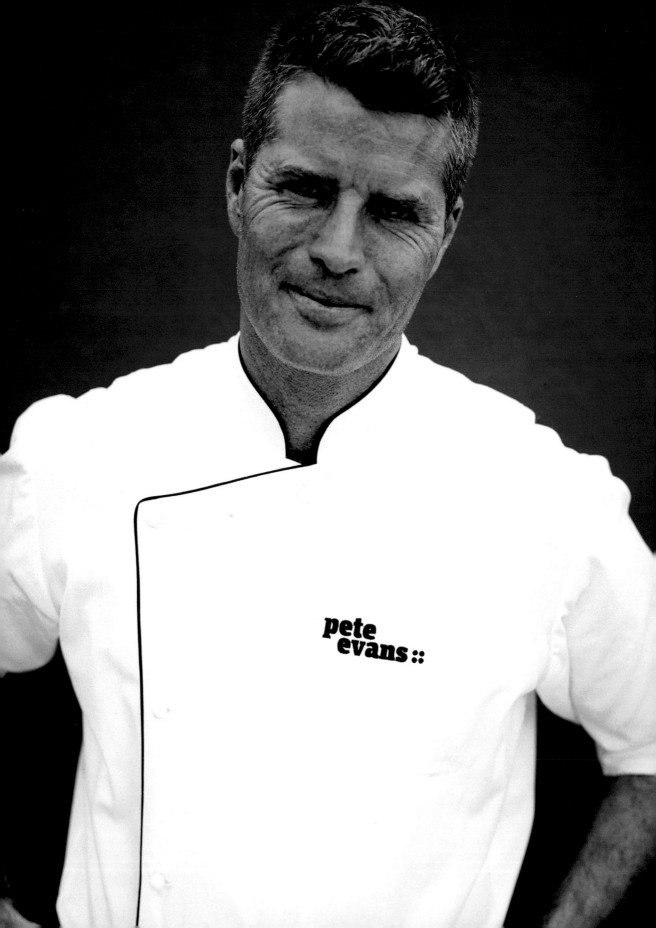

EATING AND LIVING WITH LOVE AND LAUGHTER

I love food! I love the effortless way it brings people together, its ability to create treasured memories, and, most of all, the way it provides the foundation for a vibrant, enlightened, and nourished life. I am a chef with a solid twenty-five years of experience under my apron. Because I've put in some seriously long hours in professional kitchens, I've enjoyed great success creating numerous restaurants and cooking over a million meals with my team. But I didn't want the kitchen to be my only office, so fifteen years ago, I leapt into the extraordinary world of television and cookbooks, forging a career that enables me to share my culinary passions with the world.

I've always drawn inspiration from studying and cooking foods from cultures around the globe, and not long ago, I stumbled across what many consider the oldest approach to cooking. This exciting, wholesomely traditional, affordable, attainable, and nutritionally dense way of enjoying food appealed to both my intellect and my taste buds and resonated with me more than any other dietary regimen I have ever encountered. Since then, it has guided my life and my family's lives in the most incredible, new direction, and it has opened our hearts, minds, and mouths to a wonderful lifestyle. That cooking style — you guessed it — is Paleo!

Not one to do things by halves, I threw myself into thoroughly researching the Paleo way of life — which omits refined sugars, legumes, grains, and most dairy from the daily diet — and then adopting it with vigour. As both a longtime chef and a certified health coach, I feel that I am well equipped to speak on nutrition and diet,

so my journey is now directed towards sharing my experiences and knowledge with others.

I realize that nowadays everybody is busy. I know that because I'm one of those busy people. That means that I must make it as easy as possible for you to become as healthy, strong, and happy as you can without spending loads of time, effort, or money to get there. I also know that once you start making these changes, the difference in the way you feel will inspire you to go all the way and make the Paleo lifestyle a permanent part of your life.

From the very start, I want the Paleo approach to be a totally positive experience for you. In other words, it has to be a party, not a chore. You need to see it as packed with gifts and rewards, not as weird or deprived. Toward that end, let's begin with ten things you need to know about Paleo, to help you fully understand the concept.

1. The cave is optional.

There is no need to be put off by the terms Paleolithic, primal, caveman, or Stone Age. Although many of the principles of this way of eating and living come from our hunter-gatherer ancestors, the approach I have taken is backed up by respected contemporary scientific research, common sense, and what has worked for me. (A great book to read for more information is Nora Gedgaudas's *Primal Body, Primal Mind*.) The thing is, the Paleo lifestyle is not something that someone came up with recently. It takes ideas about what made our ancestors healthy and strong survivors and adapts them to twenty-first-century life. I prefer to call what I do Paleo because that's how it was introduced to me, but you can call it what you like. The name is not important, but the next nine points are.

2. It is a way of life, not a gimmick or a diet.

There's much more to Paleo than a list of food you can or cannot eat. It's also about where that food comes from, how it's prepared, and when and how you eat it. Paleo covers how you drink, move, sleep, breathe, work, relax. In other words, it is about every aspect of life. And it's all good news.

3. Why do it?

So what's the attraction? Where's the need for Paleo? For most of us, modern life is not doing us any favours. Too many of us are inactive, sitting at desks, working on computers for most of the day, and often highly stressed. We don't get enough sleep and then reach for caffeinated, sugary drinks to keep us going through the day and for glasses of wine to wind us down at night. The food we eat is too often highly processed, and good nutrition is abandoned for the sake of convenience. For those of us who do exercise, it's invariably in a crowded room with no sunlight and with recycled air.

Sadly, too many of us in this technologically advanced era end up overweight, exhausted, stressed, and sick. And we reach for pills to fix our problems with blood pressure, digestion, blood-sugar levels, metabolism, and every other effect of our inflammation-creating and cancer-causing diet and lifestyle.

4. What to eat and drink.

My approach to Paleo is to eat whole, unprocessed foods. I advocate nose-to-tail eating and choose 100% organic, humanely raised, pasture-fed-and-finished meats and organs, which are sustainable as a food supply and healthiest for the body and the planet. I also choose wild-caught seafood from unpolluted waters; free-range poultry and pork (with no hormones or antibiotics); wild game (if available); organically grown produce, nuts, and seeds; and healthy sources of natural fats. I'm a huge fan of eating fermented food daily to keep my gut happy. Although I don't eat dairy, some people's versions of Paleo allow for specific kinds, such as full-fat natural yoghurt, certain cheeses, and raw butter from cows or goats raised on a natural diet.

When it comes to portion sizes and creating a meal, everyone goes about it differently, but here is my approach: a moderate portion of animal protein per serving (depending on how your body feels) with most of the meal made up of liberal amounts of fibrous vegetables and greens (raw, lightly cooked, and/or cultured), nuts, seeds, eggs (if tolerated), and as much natural fat as is needed to satisfy the appetite and support the healthiest brain and nervous system. Herbs and spices can be used liberally in cooking not only to add amazing flavour but also to contribute health benefits, such as polyphenols (antioxidants) that may help protect against common chronic conditions like diabetes and coronary disease. Including a small amount of seasonal fruit occasionally is purely optional.

What you drink is also important. My family and I prefer filtered water. I typically drink 3 to 4 quarts (3 to 4 litres) each day, 1 quart (1 litre) on waking and then the remainder between meals. I try not to drink during meals, as I want

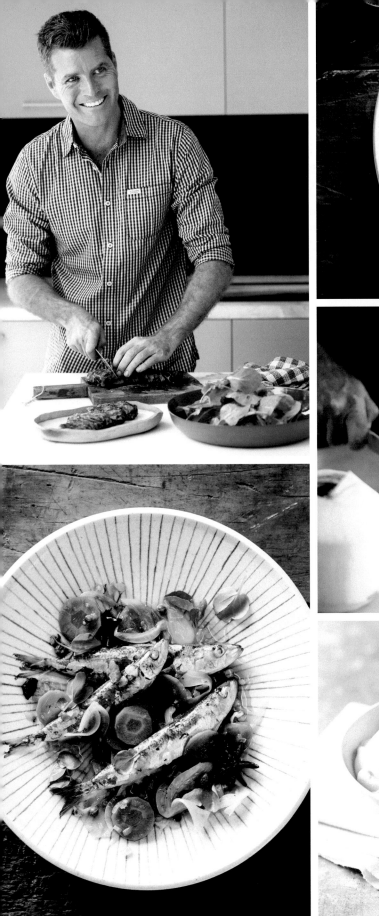
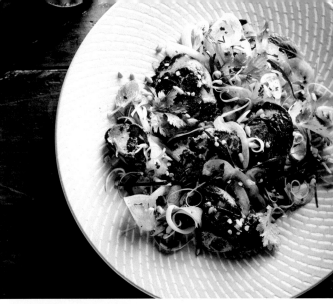
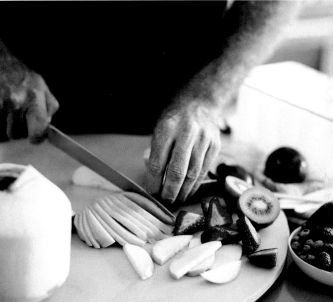
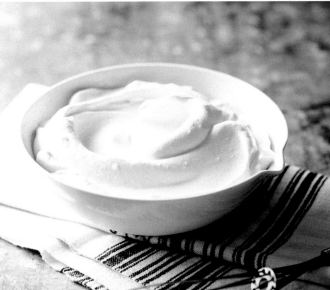

my stomach enzymes to do the work they are meant to do, which is to break down food. But if you need to drink when you're eating, take only small sips. To ensure a night of uninterrupted sleep, I tend not to drink anything after dinner except perhaps a cup of herbal tea. Look for a quality water filter for your home that eliminates unwanted chemicals, such as chlorine and fluoride, from the taps and adds back in minerals.

Fresh coconut water is an ideal treat, as are the drink recipes in this book (see pages 192 to 200). Steer clear of coffee or limit your intake because — as we all know — it is addictive and a stimulant. Also, select your herbal teas with care, as some have a diuretic effect. Avoid any beverage that has sugar in it, such as soft drinks or sports or energy drinks. Finally, limit alcohol or eliminate it altogether. If you opt for the former, source it from an organic supplier.

5. What not to eat.

Your diet will probably look very different when you eat Paleo, but don't panic. I am giving you lots of options and dozens of great recipes in this book, so you won't ever feel like you are missing out. Eliminating grains, legumes, refined sugars, and conventional dairy products still leaves plenty to celebrate, and you'll feel a lot better, too.

I make a conscious choice not to consume any animal that has lived an inhumane life on a diet it wasn't designed to eat, such as caged chickens or grain-fed cattle. I seek out dedicated farmers and anglers who offer meats, poultry, and seafood from animals that have lived a stress-free life on a natural diet. I try to eat nose-to-tail, which means I am always using different cuts and also including offal in my diet, as you will discover in my recipes. I also avoid non-organic produce, GMOs, and processed foods.

As I noted earlier, some people adapt the Paleo approach to suit their cooking and lifestyle. For example, strict Paleo followers allow no dairy with the exception of ghee (see page 7), which is basically pure fat and a much better option than trans fats. Even though I don't eat legumes, which is in keeping with Paleo principles, I do

use organic, GMO-free tamari (wheat-free soy), and miso in very small quantities in a few of my recipes because they are fermented. But people who don't want to touch soy at all can switch to coconut aminos or sugar-free fish sauce for flavouring (see page 8).

My advice is to change to Paleo slowly so that your body and mind can adapt. I would look at eliminating refined sugars from your diet for a month to start, then move on to wheat and other grains, and then to dairy if you choose. Your body might go into a detoxification state during which you feel tired and lethargic, and you may even get a bit sick, so just be mindful and aware that this is part of the journey. After a while, you will become stronger and healthier, and the foods that used to control you will no longer have power over you.

6. We're not fat and carb haters!

Not all fats are evil. In fact, some fats are essential for good health. The same is true of carbohydrates. Unfortunately, we have been taught to be afraid of animal fats and to eat lots of grains, which can exacerbate health problems.

People need a relatively high amount of good fat, which is actually better for us and easier to digest than the carbs we get from bread and pasta. These friendly fats come courtesy of olive, macadamia, and coconut oils; coconut milk; avocados; butter and ghee (clarified butter); grass-fed meat; oily fish; and nuts and seeds.

When you eat Paleo, you get plenty of good carbs from vegetables and fruits. This cuts out the problem carbs, which are the grains and refined sugars that can cause insulin resistance, digestive problems, and inflammation.

7. Find balance with omega fatty acids.

Many people's eyes glaze over when I start talking about the ratio of omega-3 to omega-6 fatty acids in our diet, but understanding what these fatty acids do is important for good health. Put simply, we should reduce the number of omega-6 fatty acids in our diet because they cause inflammation. That's why refined seed-based oils and grain-fed meats are off the menu. On the menu, because of their anti-inflammatory qualities, are omega-3s, which are found in oily fish, seafood, fish oil, linseed oil, and grass-fed meats.

8. Breathe deeply and move often, outdoors, and with others.

By not breathing properly, you are robbing your body of essential oxygen and vital energy. I do daily breathing exercises that are a simple but extremely effective way of oxygenating the body and that get me ready to start moving and fulfil my potential.

Paleo people are always on the move: they like doing a range of exercises, such as resistance training, CrossFit, swimming, stand-up paddling, yoga, walking, sprinting and hiking, and getting plenty of vitamin D while having fun in the sun with others. Play is important, and strength and fitness come with walking long distances and lifting heavy things with correct technique. Any sport or movement that you love to include in your life is encouraged.

9. Restore your rest and bliss.

Increase your sleep time – eight hours a night as often as you can do it – and you will get rid of chronic, ongoing stress. Paleo sleep is peaceful sleep, without sound, lights, and distractions to disturb it, and no digital interference in the hour leading up to it.

Little bursts of stress, before an exam or job interview, for example, are great performance enhancers. It's the prolonged and relentless stress that never lets up, day after day, week after week, month after month, that has a profoundly negative effect on a person's mood, memory, weight, immune system, blood pressure, sex drive, and fertility. With more sleep and less stress, you will see improvements in all those areas.

10. Learn lots and think positively.

Paleo energy is as much mental as it is physical. The incredibly positive differences a Paleo lifestyle can make depend heavily on the thoughts you're having and the words you use to express them. Instead of saying, 'I can't have cake', bring meaning to your decision and think, 'I choose not to have cake made from those ingredients. It makes all the difference.' (And you can still sometimes have cake; see page 167.)

Grow your mind along with your health and continue learning and searching for knowledge, improving and stimulating your mind, and stretching your horizons. Meeting new people, going to places you've never been before, and thinking in new ways will dramatically enhance the effects of your healthful eating and exercise.

With all that said, you're ready to let your mind, body, and taste buds be astonished by some exceptional ways to prepare what Mother Nature graciously provides us. Outstanding food and renewed health are only a few pages away!

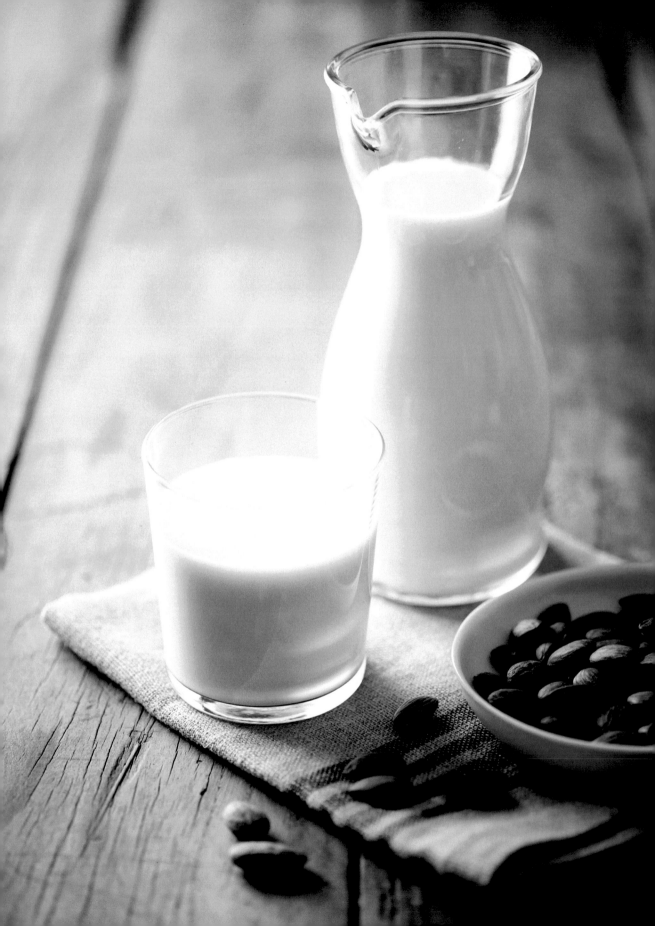

ABOUT INGREDIENTS

This section is devoted to ingredients I've included in my recipes. I know that some ingredients I use are not eaten by everyone because of individual differences in Paleo diets, so to make the recipes acceptable to the broadest range of cooks, I have tried to offer an alternative ingredient whenever possible. No matter which ingredients you choose, always select the highest-quality, organic, and sustainable products you can find and afford.

ACTIVATED NUTS. Nuts are a fantastically healthful snack, loaded with protein, good fats, fibre, and important minerals like zinc, magnesium, and calcium. However, it's best to activate your nuts before eating them or using them in recipes. This is easily done by soaking them in filtered water and then drying or toasting them. This simple process, which I have suggested throughout the book, releases the enzyme inhibitors and phytic acid present in the nuts, which means our bodies can more easily absorb all of the great nutrients they contain. When nuts are not activated, it is difficult for our digestive system to break down and absorb these beneficial elements.

EGGS. The best, most delicious eggs come from organically fed, pasture-raised chickens that are allowed to roam outside freely in the sunshine, eat insects and plants, and have healthier and happier lives than their cage-trapped cousins. These eggs taste better, have stronger shells, are less runny, and have firmer and brighter yolks. They also contain less cholesterol and saturated fat and have higher levels of vitamins A, E, and D; protein; beta-carotene; and omega-3 fatty acids than eggs from caged birds.

GHEE. This is the pure, clarified butterfat that remains after milk solids and water are removed from butter, which means that ghee is essentially dairy-free. It has a pleasantly rich, nutty taste and is high in vitamins A, D, E, and K_2. When sourced from grass-fed cows, it contains naturally occurring CLA (conjugated linoleic acid) as well as omega-3 and other essential fatty acids. It is an ideal ingredient in cooking and baking, but because not everyone following a Paleo diet uses it, I always offer another choice in my recipes. One of my favourite alternative sources of fat is coconut oil, which is extracted from the flesh of mature coconuts and is believed to have numerous health benefits.

MAPLE SYRUP. Like raw honey, maple syrup is a healthful alternative to sugar. It is packed with anti-inflammatory and antioxidant compounds and important essential nutrients like zinc, iron, calcium, and potassium. Be sure to choose 100 percent pure maple syrup (made from boiling down the sap of the maple tree), rather than maple-flavoured syrup. As with any sweetener, it should be used in moderation. Consuming too much can lead to weight gain, unhealthy blood levels of fat and cholesterol, and high blood pressure.

MEAT AND POULTRY. This is an easy one: if you eat meat and poultry, always seek out the best quality possible. At the minimum, that means whatever you buy must be chemical- and hormone-free. Whenever possible, purchase grass-fed, pasture-raised, and organic products from a local, environmentally aware farm or shop. They might cost a little more, but it's worth it for your health and the health of the environment. You can cut costs by not eating big portions and by choosing cuts that braise beautifully or organ meats, such as liver, kidney, and heart, that offer a rich mix of nutrients. And be sure to use the bones to make nutrient-dense stocks.

QUINOA. Although quinoa is technically not a grain, some Paleo followers choose not to consume it because it packs a punch in the carb stakes and, like many grains, can irritate the gut. The jury is out on whether or not to include it in a Paleo diet. I tend to keep it off the menu, but I know people who do eat it, so do as your body dictates.

RAW HONEY. Pure, unheated, unpasteurized, and unprocessed, raw honey comes in both liquid and solid form. It preserves all of the natural vitamins, enzymes, phytonutrients, antioxidants, and other nutritional elements that your body needs and is perfect for adding a little sweetness to savoury foods, hot and cold drinks, and desserts. Consuming too much can lead to weight gain, unhealthy blood levels of fat and cholesterol, and high blood pressure.

SALT. I use pure unprocessed salt, such as sea salt and Himalayan rock salt, for everyday cooking. Mineral-rich Himalayan salt, sometimes labelled Himalayan pink salt, is one of my favourites. Tens of millions of years old and free of the toxins and pollutants that plague many other types of ocean salt, it boasts a translucent pink colour and is often sold in crystal form, though finely ground Himalayan salt is available. Many different minerals and elements are naturally found in the salt: sodium, iron, magnesium, calcium, and copper are present in trace amounts, for example, with the iron delivering the beautiful pink colour. On the flip side, I avoid traditional iodized salt, which is heavily processed, bleached, and contains aluminium.

SEAFOOD. It's an excellent source of protein, vitamins, minerals, and omega-3 fatty acids. As a chef who loves cooking and eating seafood, and as an enthusiastic fisherman, surfer, and father, I care passionately about the future health of our oceans. Our seas connect every continent and shape every coast. They control our climate and produce much of the oxygen we breathe. It's more important than ever to choose sustainable fish and shellfish and to put a stop to the overfishing and pollution of our oceans and other waterways. According to the Food and Agricultural Organization of the United Nations (UNFAO), more than 1 billion people rely on seafood as their main source of protein, and more than 200 million livelihoods depend on the seafood industry. Healthy fish stocks and marine ecosystems are not only vital for the well-being of the world's oceans but also for the health of the world's people and their economy.

By choosing seafood that comes from sustainable fisheries, you are helping to protect the marine environment and safeguard future seafood supplies. But selecting sustainable seafood can be difficult. One way to identify certified sustainable seafood is to look for the blue ecolabel of the Marine Stewardship Council (MSC). Seafood that displays the label can be traced from plate or packaged product all the way back to a certified sustainable fishery. Other organizations, such as Seafood Watch, Friend of the Sea, and the World Wildlife Fund, are excellent resources as well.

TAMARI. A sauce made from whole, fermented soybeans, this is similar to soy sauce but is richer and less salty and contains no wheat, so it's gluten-free. It is not strictly Paleo, of course, because it is made from soybeans, but it is fermented and I only use it in small amounts. You will see tamari throughout the book, but if you choose not to use it in your diet, a great alternative is coconut aminos, which has a similar flavour but is slightly less salty and contains a higher level of amino acids, vitamins B and C, and various minerals.

One of the biggest trends in culinary and nutrition circles is fermented, or cultured, foods. Fermentation is what gives kefir its tartness and miso its umami flair. In addition to occupying a special niche in cuisine, these traditional cultured foods are some of the most nutrient-dense foods available to us.

POWER OF FERMENTED FOODS

What exactly do fermented foods do for you and why are they such a hot topic? Fermentation preserves nutrients, vitamins, and enzymes in foods. Not only do fermented foods give you a vitamin boost but also, through fermentation, they create enzymes, organic acids, and vitamins such as B and K that are not naturally found in the original food. The production of enzymes is especially important because as you age, your supply of enzymes, which help the body utilize the nutrients in food, naturally decreases.

Fermented foods are amazing for your gut, where approximately 70 percent of your immune system is located. Not only do they strengthen your immune system, improve digestion, and eliminate toxins, but they can also restore the proper balance of bacteria in your gut – helpful for anyone with food intolerances – and make nutrients more available to the body, so that they can be absorbed more readily. If that isn't enough, cultured vegetables are rich in lactobacilli and lactic acids. These bacteria and their by-products beneficially alter the pH of the intestines, which in turn helps prevent the overgrowth of unfriendly bacteria, mould, and yeasts like candida.

Finally, fermenting food helps to preserve it for longer periods of time without the use of modern chemical preservatives. Culturing your own food is relatively inexpensive and far cheaper than buying probiotics, plus homemade cultured foods will add great flavour to your meals.

———————————————————————————

When fermenting foods, I always follow a few simple guidelines:

1. Use filtered water when making cultured foods, as the chlorine found in tap water inhibits the growth of the beneficial bacteria that you trying to encourage in lacto-fermentation.

2. Use an unrefined sea salt. Table salt contains iodine and an anticaking agent that interfere with the process of fermentation by neutralizing the necessary yeasts.

3. Be sure that the vessel you use is capable of creating a hermetically sealed anaerobic environment (meaning without oxygen). The ideal fermenting jar is made of lead-free glass, so that no chemicals will leach into

This enables the lactic acid bacteria to multiply and thrive in an oxygen-free climate, yielding a higher probiotic count. Oxygen neutralizes the lactic acid bacteria and you end up losing the benefits, plus it can lead to the growth of moulds, unfriendly yeasts, and pathogenic bacteria.

Despite being popular, open-air systems with loose-fitting lids, such as Mason jars or stoneware crocks, are better suited to making vinegar and kombucha, both of which require an aerobic process (with oxygen) to create an acetic acid fermentation rather than a lactic acid one.

BREAKFAST

13

hazelnut & banana
pancakes

14

sweet potato röstis with
poached eggs, spinach,
avocado & smoked salmon

17

coconut vanilla yoghurt

18

soft-boiled eggs with
salmon roe & asparagus

21

stir-fried beef with basil,
chilli & fried eggs

22

seed & nut bread

25

asparagus with soft-boiled
eggs, capers & bone
marrow broth

26

muesli & berry parfait
with coconut cream

29

prawn omelette with dashi
broth & asian greens

30

liquorice root sausages with
fried eggs & greens

33

courgette & fennel fritters

34

nasi goreng

37

scrambled eggs with smoked
trout, kale & horseradish

38

black chia seed puddings
with nuts, figs & dates

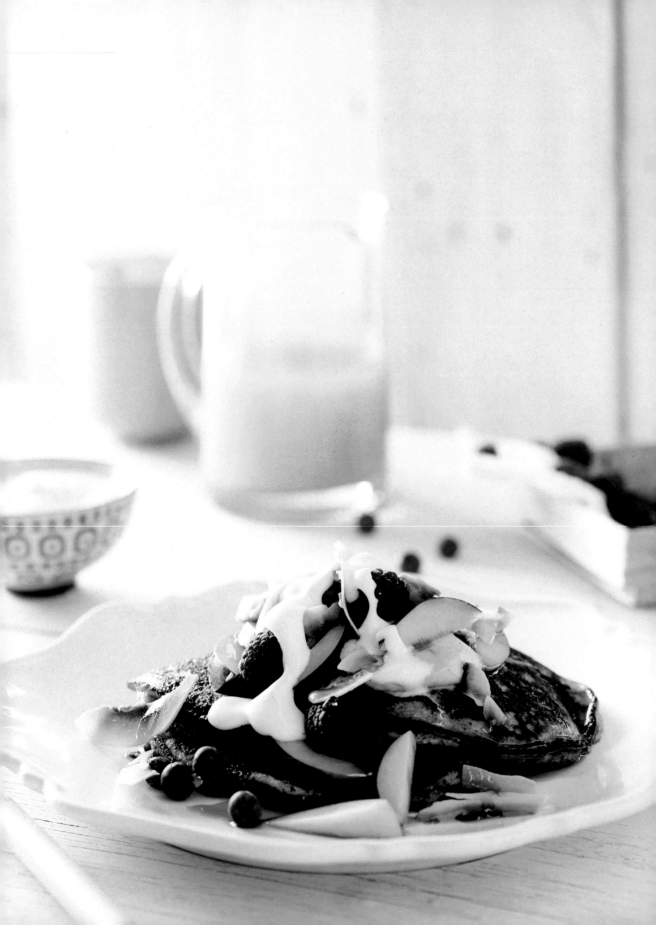

My family and I enjoy pancakes every once in a while, but they are not the most nutritious breakfast (sautéed greens will always win out as the better choice). This recipe doesn't contain all of the typical pancake ingredients like wheat flour, refined sugars, or dairy, so it's a more acceptable choice than the standard pancake recipes out there. And, if you feel the need to add a side of greens and some bacon, be my guest! You can also add other fruit to the mixture besides those mentioned here. Keep the pancakes small in size, and don't get distracted while cooking them to ensure they don't burn.

HAZELNUT & BANANA PANCAKES

SERVES 2

4 eggs

6 tbsp (120 ml) almond milk (page 192) or other nut milk

2 tbsp raw honey

¼ tsp vanilla powder

1 cup (100 g) ground hazelnuts, activated (page 209)

1½ tbsp coconut flour

2 tsp baking powder

Pinch of ground cinnamon

Coconut oil or ghee, for cooking, plus more to serve

2 bananas, sliced

to serve
Raw honey or maple syrup (optional)

Freshly squeezed lemon juice

Fresh fruit, such as berries and sliced stone fruit

Toasted coconut flakes

Coconut cream

In a small bowl, whisk the eggs for about 2 minutes, or until frothy. Mix in the almond milk, honey, and vanilla powder.

In a larger bowl, combine the ground hazelnuts, coconut flour, baking powder, cinnamon, and a pinch of sea salt. Stir the wet mixture into the dry ingredients until the coconut flour is fully incorporated.

Grease a large frying pan with a little coconut oil and heat over medium heat. Ladle a few tbsp of the batter into the pan for each pancake, spread out slightly with the back of a spoon, and add some sliced banana. The pancakes should be about 3 inches (7.5 cm) in diameter and fairly thick. Cook for a few minutes, until the top dries out slightly and the bottom starts to brown. Flip and cook for an additional 40 seconds, or until cooked through.

Serve hot with ghee; a drizzle of honey or maple syrup, if using; and a squeeze of lemon juice, accompanied by fresh fruit, toasted coconut flakes, and coconut cream.

Enjoying avocado for breakfast is what my body loves! I usually eat an avocado or two a day because it increases my healthy fat and calorie intake without seriously increasing my protein or carbohydrate intake. Avocados are rich in monounsaturated fat, which our bodies burn as energy. They're low in fructose, which is ideal because they don't jack up insulin levels, and they provide plenty of health-boosting nutrients like fibre, potassium (more than twice the amount found in a banana), vitamins B and E, and folic acid. This is a fantastic recipe that's easy to whip up. And if you are focusing on weight loss, it's even great without the sweet potato *rösti*.

SWEET POTATO RÖSTIS
WITH POACHED EGGS, SPINACH, AVOCADO & SMOKED SALMON
SERVES 4

sweet potato rösti
1⅓ lb (600 g) sweet potatoes, peeled and grated

2 eggs

1 tbsp chopped fresh flat-leaf parsley

2 to 3 tbsp coconut oil, duck fat, or ghee

poached eggs
2 tbsp raw apple cider vinegar

4 eggs

1 clove garlic, finely chopped

2 large handfuls of baby spinach

2 tbsp (30 g) salmon roe

8 slices smoked wild salmon or other smoked fish

1 avocado, peeled, pitted, and sliced

8 caper berries, halved

¼ bunch of dill, stems removed and sprigs torn into small pieces

Lemon wedges

To make the sweet potato *röstis*, squeeze all of the excess moisture out of the grated sweet potatoes. Combine the sweet potatoes with the eggs and parsley and stir until combined. Season with sea salt and freshly cracked black pepper.

Heat a large nonstick frying pan over medium-high heat and add 1 tbsp of the oil. When the oil is melted and hot, place about 2 tbsp of the mixture to form patties in the pan. Cook until the bottom is golden, 2 to 3 minutes. Turn over and cook the other side until golden. Do this in batches if necessary, adding more oil as needed. Keep the *röstis* warm on a baking sheet in a low oven.

Meanwhile, poach the eggs, add the vinegar and some salt to a saucepan of boiling water, then reduce the heat to medium-low so the water is just simmering. Crack 1 egg into a cup. Using a wooden spoon or whisk, stir the simmering water in one direction to form a whirlpool and drop the egg into the centre. Repeat with the remaining 3 eggs. Cook for 3 minutes, or until cooked to your liking. Using a slotted spoon, remove the eggs and place on a paper towel to soak up the excess water.

To finish, add a touch more oil to the frying pan and add the garlic. Cook until just fragrant, about 1 minute. Add the spinach and cook until the spinach is wilted, 1 to 2 minutes. Season with salt and pepper. Drain the spinach on a paper towel or kitchen towel to remove any liquid (to keep each *rösti* nice and crispy when you pop the spinach on it).

To serve, divide the sweet potato *röstis* among four serving plates. Top the *röstis* with wilted spinach, then a poached egg and some salmon roe. Divide the smoked salmon, avocado, caper berries, dill, and lemon wedges among the plates. Sprinkle each with salt and pepper.

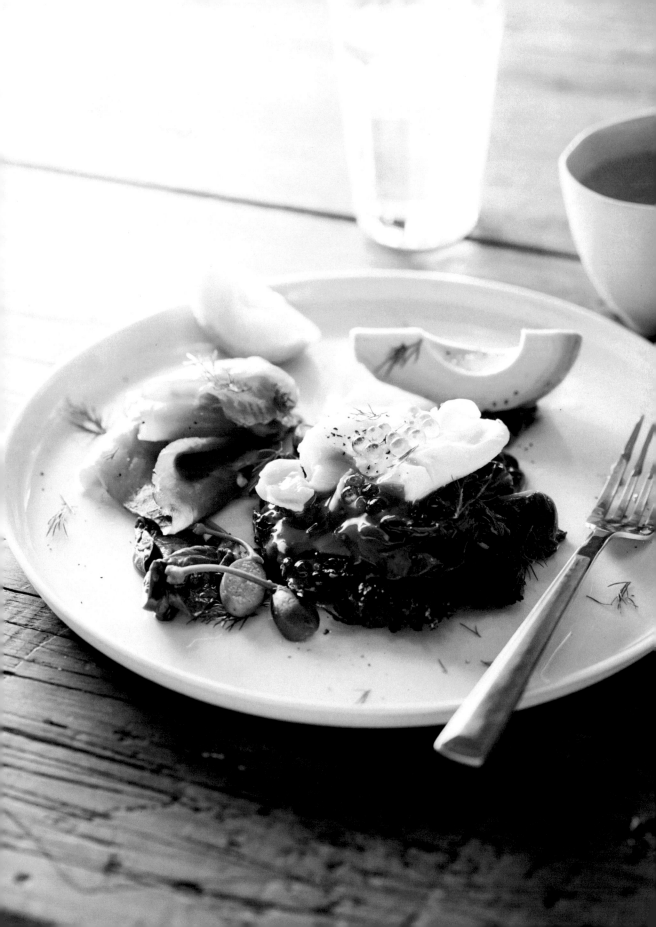

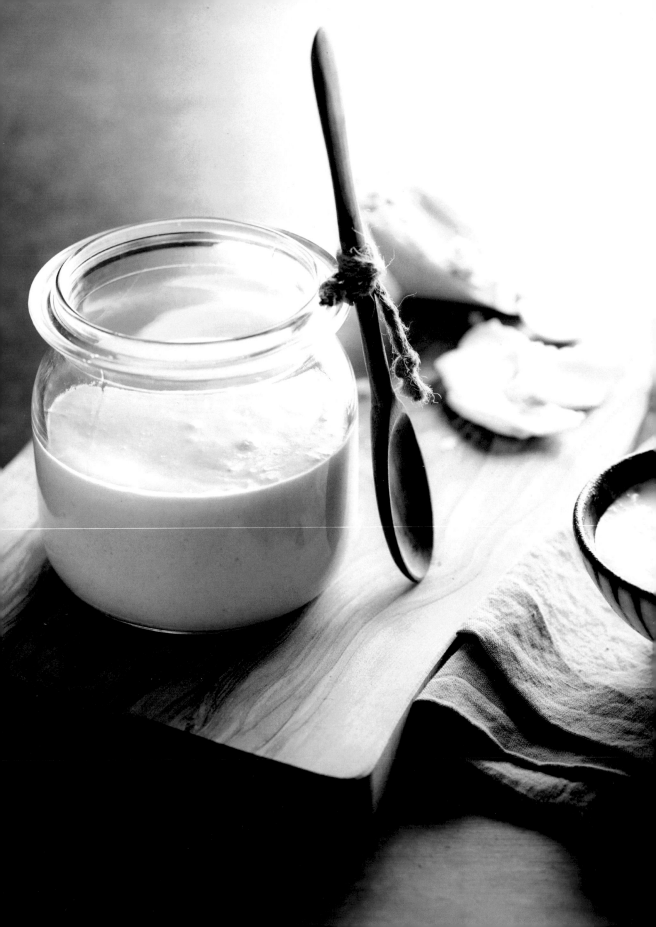

My dear Mum fed me cow's milk yoghurt pretty much every day of my early childhood, neither of us realizing that I was lactose intolerant. She thought the fact that I was constantly sneezing was due to my weak immune system. I haven't consumed dairy in large quantities now for more than twenty years, and my health is a lot better for it. This recipe for creamy yoghurt is made with coconut flesh and sweetened with the sweetener of your choice. This yoghurt is loaded with healthy bacteria and is delicious either on its own, with a sprinkling of fresh berries, or served with some crunchy Paleo muesli (page 26).

COCONUT VANILLA YOGHURT

MAKES ABOUT 2½ cups (600 ml)

4 young green coconuts

2 tbsp lemon juice

Seeds of 1 to 2 scraped vanilla beans (or substitute ½ tsp vanilla powder)

Maple syrup, raw honey, or green leaf stevia powder

2 probiotic capsules

Open the tops of the coconuts and pour out the coconut water into a measuring cup. Remove the coconut flesh out of the shells and roughly chop. Add the coconut flesh, ½ cup (125 ml) coconut water, the lemon juice, vanilla bean seeds, and sweetener to taste. Blend until smooth and creamy. Depending on the consistency you prefer, you can add more coconut water. Open your probiotic capsules, pour into the blender, and give it one final quick whirl.

Pour the mixture into a 1-quart (1 L) glass jar, cover with the lid, and allow it to sit for at least 5 hours or up to 12 hours at room temperature so that the bacteria can proliferate (and convert sugars to lactic acid to make yoghurt). The longer you leave it, the tangier it becomes. Cover and store it in the fridge for up to 1 week.

I'm an egg lover. I eat two to four eggs a day, using raw eggs in my smoothies and creamy yolks in homemade mayo, or I enjoy them simply scrambled, poached, fried, soft-boiled, or in an omelette. And if I can get my hands on duck eggs, I'm a seriously happy guy. Eggs truly are one of nature's super foods, and many say they are better for you than multivitamins. This recipe is a family favourite in our home. The kids actually voted this as their all-time number one breakfast; and yes, they love the salmon roe. Throw in fresh asparagus and sprouted seed bread for some good old traditional dipping.

SOFT-BOILED EGGS
WITH SALMON ROE & ASPARAGUS
SERVES 4

dressing
3 tbsp extra virgin olive oil or macadamia nut oil

½ shallot, finely chopped

1 tbsp raw apple cider vinegar

1 tsp finely chopped fresh flat-leaf parsley

½ tsp fermented mustard (page 206)

8 eggs

14 oz (400 g) green and/or white asparagus, trimmed and halved lengthwise

⅓ cup (80 g) salmon roe

Seed & Nut Bread (page 22)

To make the dressing, mix together the oil, shallot, vinegar, parsley, and mustard. Season with sea salt and freshly cracked black pepper and set aside.

Put the eggs in a large saucepan and cover with cold water. Bring to a boil and cook to your liking (4 minutes for soft yolks).

Meanwhile, cook the asparagus in boiling salted water until tender but still slightly crisp, about 1 minute, then drain. Toss the asparagus with the dressing and season with salt and pepper.

To serve, divide the asparagus spears among four plates. Remove the tops from the soft-boiled eggs and set the eggs in egg cups. Spoon 1 tbsp of salmon roe on top of each egg and finish with cracked pepper. Serve with toasted bread.

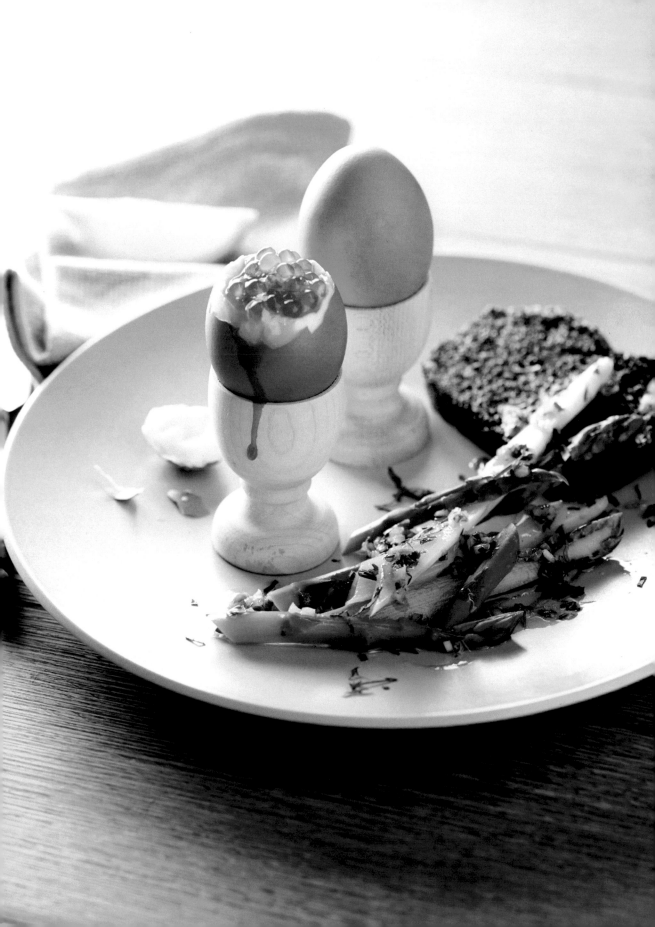

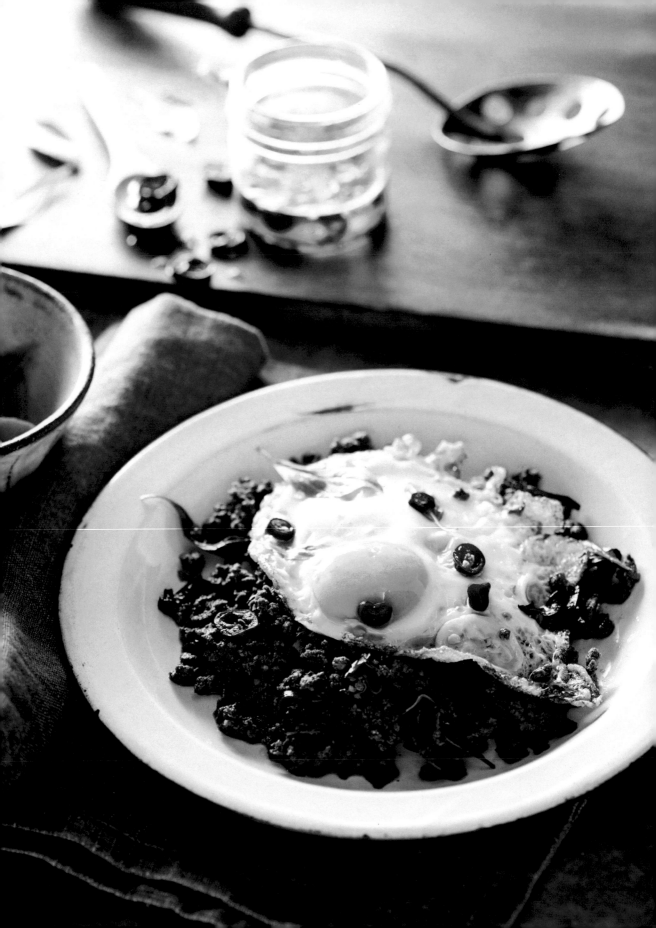

This dish is inspired by a classic Thai street food dish and is meant to pack quite a punch, so don't be shy with the chillies if you can handle the heat. You can use any type of ground meat for this dish — even ground chicken for something different — but it works especially well with anything that has a high fat content. Thai basil, a sweet purple basil, is one of the most exciting herbs to add to your cooking repertoire because it has the most heavenly aroma. If you can't get your hands on it, substitute Italian basil or fresh coriander, and the dish will still be super tasty. Sautéed spinach, kale, okra, or broccoli florets would be a great, healthy addition to this dish.

STIR-FRIED BEEF
WITH BASIL, CHILLI & FRIED EGGS

SERVES 2

hot and sour sauce
⅓ cup (80 ml) fish sauce

Juice of 2 limes

4 bird's eye chillies, thinly sliced

1 clove garlic, finely chopped

1 tsp peeled and grated fresh ginger

1 tsp raw honey (optional)

Fresh coriander, chopped

stir-fry
3 tbsp coconut oil, plus more if needed

2 eggs

2 fresh red chillies, sliced

3 cloves garlic, finely chopped

10½ oz (300 g) minced beef

½ cup (125 ml) chicken stock (page 202)

1 tbsp fish sauce, or to taste

1 tbsp wheat-free tamari or coconut aminos (optional)

1 tsp raw honey (optional)

¼ tsp Chinese five-spice powder

2 large handfuls of fresh Thai basil leaves

To make the sauce, combine the fish sauce, lime juice, bird's eye chillies, garlic, ginger, and honey, if using, in a small bowl; mix well and set aside. For best results, make this at least 1 hour or up to 1 day in advance; the longer you leave it, the stronger the sauce will be.

To make the stir-fry, heat a wok or a large frying pan over medium-high heat. Add 1 tbsp of the coconut oil and swirl it around the pan. Crack one egg into the centre and fry until cooked to your liking, 1 to 2 minutes. Shake the wok gently to prevent the egg from sticking. Carefully lift out the egg with a spatula and place on a plate and keep warm. Repeat with the other egg, adding a little more oil if needed.

Return the wok to high heat. Add the remaining 2 tbsp of coconut oil and swirl it around the wok. Add the chillies and garlic and cook until fragrant, 1 minute. Add the beef and stir-fry until brown, 2 minutes. Add the chicken stock and simmer for 3 minutes. Mix in the fish sauce; tamari and honey, if using; and five-spice powder. Toss in the basil and, as soon as it is wilted, remove the wok from the heat. Season to taste with sea salt and freshly cracked black pepper.

To serve, divide the meat between two serving plates and top each with a warm fried egg. Sprinkle the hot and sour sauce with freshly chopped coriander and serve the sauce on the side to drizzle over the dish to your liking.

I know that people don't like change, and for some, the fear of giving up their daily routine of toast or sandwiches to follow a Paleo diet is a big one, especially if they are addicted to those things. There is, however, a non-addictive, healthier option than and it is nothing short of deliciously satisfying. It is a much wiser alternative than modern-day bread (even many of the gluten-free versions of bread in the supermarkets contain hidden nasties). From time to time I like to load up a slice of this hearty bread with avocado, fermented veggies, and lots of herbs.

SEED & NUT BREAD
MAKES 1 LOAF

4 tbsp sunflower seeds, activated (page 209) and chopped

4 tbsp pumpkin seeds, activated (page 209) and chopped

2 tbsp chia seeds

⅔ cup (50 g) almonds, activated (page 209) and chopped

1½ cups (155 g) ground almonds

¼ cup (25 g) LSA meal (page 209)

2 tbsp coconut flour

1 tsp baking soda

6 eggs

⅓ cup (80 ml) coconut oil, melted, plus more for greasing

1 tbsp raw honey

1 tbsp raw apple cider vinegar

Preheat the oven to 325°F (160°C gas 3). Mix the sunflower, pumpkin, and chia seeds together in a bowl; set aside 3 tbsp for sprinkling over the bread before baking. Add the chopped almonds, ground almonds, LSA meal, coconut flour, and baking soda to the remaining seeds in the bowl. Add the eggs, coconut oil, honey, vinegar, and ½ tsp sea salt and mix well until combined. Grease an 8 by 4-inch (20 by 10 cm) loaf tin with coconut oil and line with baking parchment. Pour the mixture into the tin and smooth it out evenly, then sprinkle the top with the reserved mixed seeds.

Bake for 45 to 50 minutes, or until the loaf is golden and a metal skewer inserted in the centre of the loaf comes out clean. (You will need to do the skewer test because this bread is much denser than regular bread and won't sound hollow when you tap it.)

Let the bread cool completely in the tin before turning out. Store the bread wrapped in plastic wrap in the refrigerator for up to 5 days, or in the freezer for up to 3 months.

Note: For a sweeter loaf add 6 finely chopped medjool dates along with the eggs.

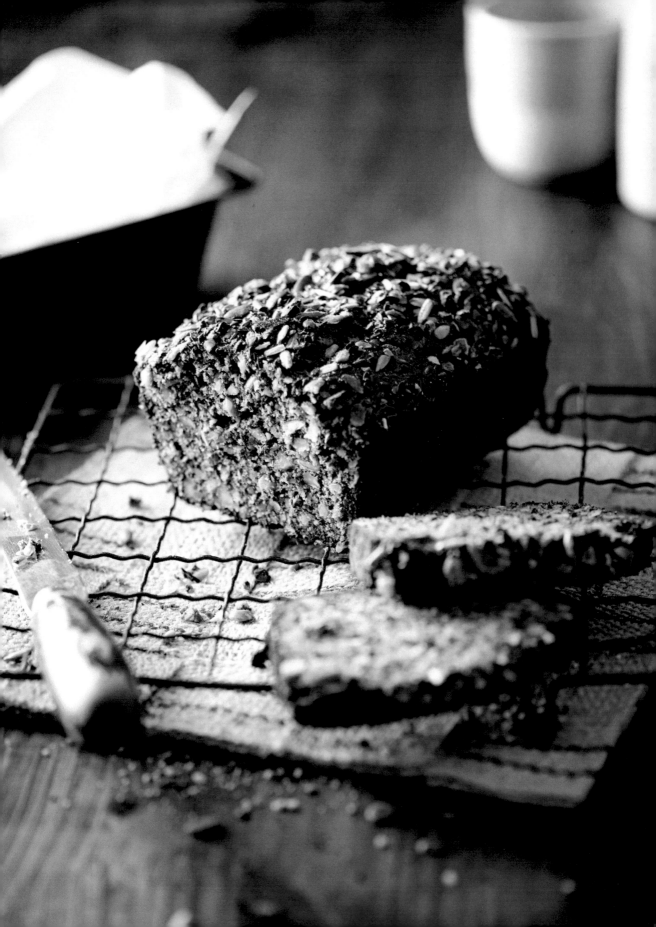

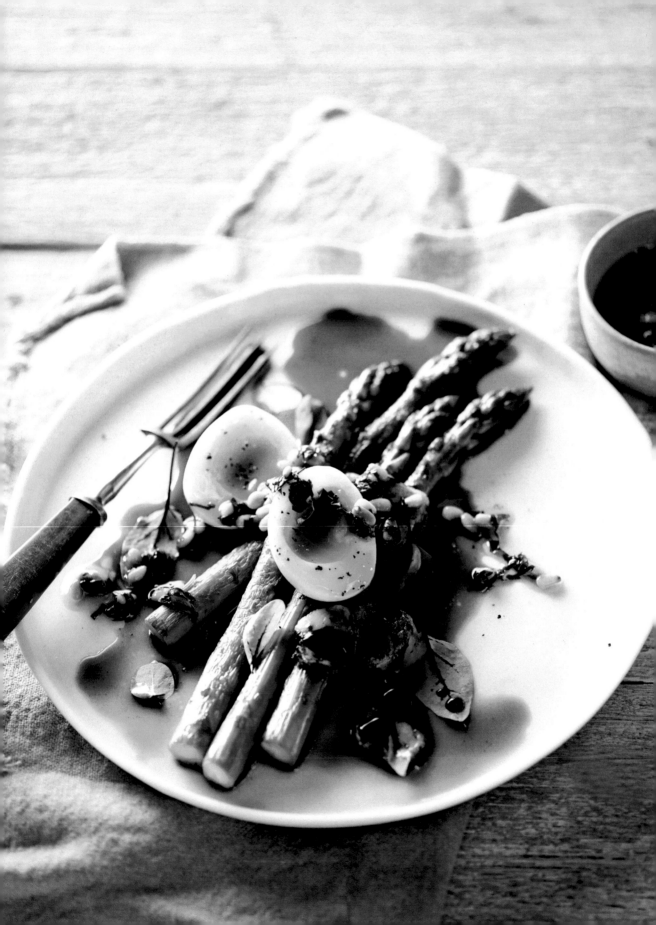

Bone marrow is a wonderfully fatty, gelatinous substance found in the core of bones. Eating it helps improve brain function, maintain healthy bones, support immune systems, and speed up the healing process from injuries and fractures. I find bone marrow extremely delicious, and it's one of my favourite ingredients to work with, not only for its taste but also for its silky richness and the unique texture it gives food. In this recipe, I have added it to a reduced stock and teamed it with asparagus, soft-boiled eggs, and capers. I find this to be wonderful dish to serve at breakfast, lunch, or dinner to bring warmth and comfort to the body.

ASPARAGUS
WITH SOFT-BOILED EGGS, CAPERS & BONE MARROW BROTH

SERVES 4

bone marrow broth

2 lb (900 g) beef marrow bones, cut into 2-inch (5 cm) pieces

4 cups (1 L) beef stock (page 203)

1 tsp raw apple cider vinegar

1 tsp chopped fresh thyme leaves

2 bunches of asparagus, trimmed

4 eggs, at room temperature

2 tbsp ghee or coconut oil, plus more as needed

2 cloves garlic, finely chopped

2 tbsp baby capers, rinsed

2 tbsp pine nuts, toasted

Sorrel, preferably red-veined

To make the bone marrow broth, pop out the marrow from the bones and slice the bone marrow into ⅓-inch (1 cm) thick pieces and set aside. Heat the stock in a saucepan over medium heat and reduce by just over half, or until 1½ cups (350 ml) remain, 15 to 20 minutes. Add the vinegar, thyme, and sea salt and freshly cracked black pepper to taste; set aside and keep warm.

Meanwhile, cook the asparagus in boiling salted water until tender but still slightly crisp, about 1 minute, then drain. Plunge in cold water to stop the cooking, then set aside until needed.

To prepare the eggs, bring a saucepan filled with water to a boil over medium heat. Turn down to a simmer, add the eggs, and cook for 4½ minutes (for soft-boiled), or until cooked to your liking. Remove with a slotted spoon and peel.

Heat a frying pan over medium heat, gently heat the ghee, then add the garlic and cook just until it starts to colour, about 1 minute. Add the asparagus, capers, and salt and pepper and cook, tossing, until the asparagus turns slightly golden, about 30 seconds.

To finish the bone marrow broth, in another frying pan over medium heat, add a little ghee and pan-fry the bone marrow for 40 seconds on each side, or until lightly brown. Drain all but 1 tbsp fat from the pan. Add the reduced stock to the bone marrow and bring to a boil, then remove from the heat.

To serve, divide the asparagus among four serving plates and spoon over the caper dressing from the pan. Cut the eggs in half lengthwise and top the asparagus with the egg halves. Garnish with pine nuts and sorrel, spoon over a good amount of bone marrow reduction, and finish with pepper over the egg.

Layered with muesli, whipped coconut cream, and berry puree, this Paleo parfait is not only a stellar breakfast dish, but it also makes a great snack or an elegant dessert. Because the muesli is relatively easy to prepare, I suggest making a large batch of it to store in an airtight container in the fridge; you can sprinkle the muesli over a scoop of your favourite Paleo ice cream or add some to your smoothies for a little extra crunch. Feel free to play around with your own additions to the muesli. Make sure that the coconut cream is super cold before beating it and look for a brand that contains no hidden nasties.

MUESLI & BERRY PARFAIT
WITH COCONUT CREAM

SERVES 4

muesli
½ cup (85 g) linseeds

¼ cup (35 g) pumpkin seeds

3 tbsp sesame seeds

½ cup (80 g) almonds, activated (page 209)

½ cup (55 g) unsweetened shredded dried coconut

1½ cups (230 g) frozen mixed berries

2½ tbsp raw honey

1 apple, grated

1 large carrot, peeled and grated

4 tbsp goji berries, soaked in ½ cup (125 ml) water for 10 minutes, then drained

1⅔ cups (375 ml) coconut cream

to serve (optional)
Cacao nibs

Fresh berries

Mint leaves

To make the muesli, preheat the oven to 350°F (180°C gas 4). Line three baking sheets with baking parchment. On one baking sheet, toast the linseeds, pumpkin seeds, and sesame seeds for about 8 to 10 minutes, until golden. On the second baking sheet, toast the almonds for 8 to 10 minutes, until lightly coloured. On the third baking sheet, toast the coconut for 2 to 3 minutes, or until lightly golden. Once the ingredients are toasted, combine in a large bowl and set aside to cool.

Meanwhile, in a medium saucepan, combine the frozen berries and 2 tbsp of the honey and slowly cook over low to medium heat, until they have a sauce-like consistency. Mash the berries up to create a puree, then set aside.

Combine the apple, carrot, and goji berries with the muesli and set aside.

Combine the coconut cream and ½ tbsp honey in the bowl of an electric mixer fitted with a whisk attachment. Whip the cream on high speed until soft peaks form, about 5 minutes.

In a parfait glass, start to layer with a couple of tbsp of the muesli mixture, then a couple of dollops of coconut cream, then the berry puree. Continue layering in the same order until you fill the glass. Repeat to fill three more glasses. If you like, finish with a sprinkle of cacao nibs, fresh berries, and mint leaves.

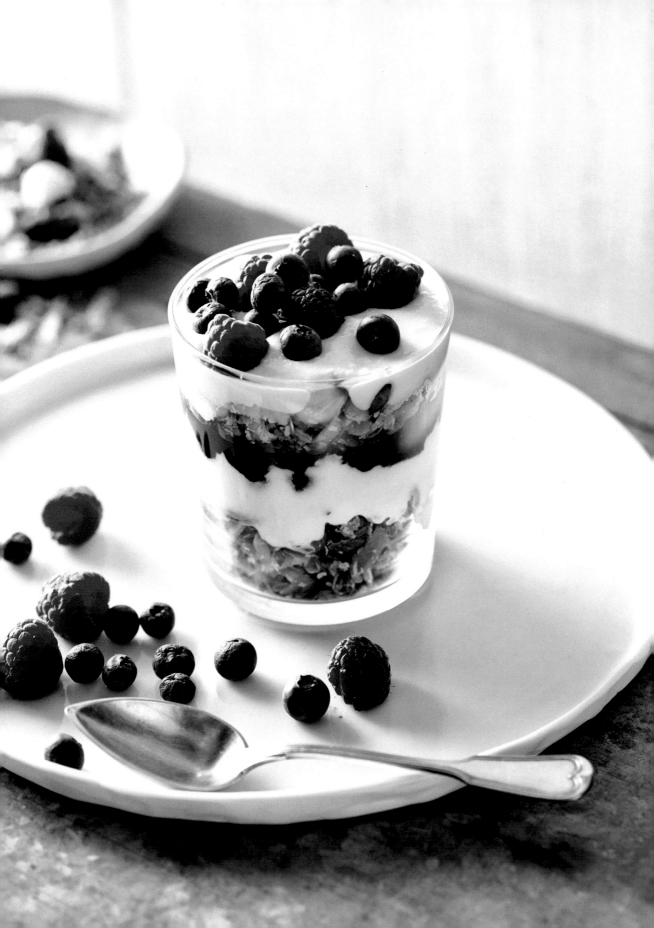

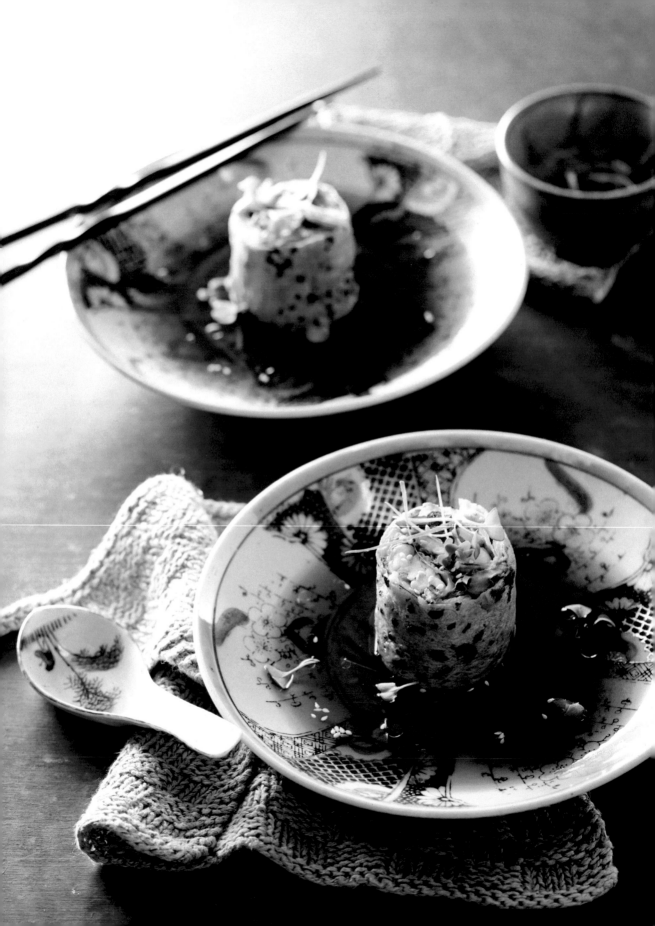

This dish looks fancy, but it's truly quite simple to make, and it works well as an impressive breakfast dish or even a light lunch or dinner. You can simplify this dish by stir-frying the ingredients first, then adding the eggs to create a delicious scramble. With a scramble, the broth is not necessary; however, adding half a cup brings a beautiful lightness to the dish. Dashi powder is made from a mix of katsuobushi, a dried fermented bonito (a type of tuna), and seaweed. It adds a lovely umami flavour, one of the five basic tastes in Japan.

PRAWN OMELETTE
WITH DASHI BROTH & ASIAN GREENS
SERVES 2

broth and vegetables
½-inch (2.5 cm) piece fresh ginger, peeled and julienned

½ fresh red chilli, halved

1 packet (1 tsp/4 g) dashi powder

1 tbsp wheat-free tamari or coconut aminos

5 oz (150 g) bok choy, choy sum, and/or Chinese broccoli, coarsely chopped

omelette
3 eggs

1 tbsp fish sauce

½ tsp raw honey

Pinch of ground turmeric

2 tbsp plus 1 tsp ghee or coconut oil

8 medium prawns, peeled and de-veined, heads and tails removed

4 shiitake mushrooms, sliced

1 spring onion, finely chopped

⅓ cup (40 g) bean sprouts

1½ tsp wheat-free tamari or coconut aminos

to serve
Bonito flakes

Black sesame seeds

Toasted sesame oil

Spring onions, pale and green parts only, thinly sliced

Asian microgreens (optional)

To make the broth, combine 2½ cups (600 ml) water, ginger, chilli, dashi powder, and tamari in a saucepan over a medium-high heat. Bring to a boil, decrease the heat to a simmer, and cook for 5 minutes. Add the vegetables to the broth and cook until tender, 10 minutes. Check for seasoning and add sea salt and freshly cracked black pepper, if needed. Strain the vegetables from the broth (reserve the broth) and place the vegetables on a paper towel to drain any excess liquid. Set the vegetables aside and keep the broth hot.

Meanwhile, mix together the eggs, fish sauce, honey, and turmeric in a bowl and set aside.

Heat a frying pan over medium-high heat and add 1 tbsp of the ghee. When the ghee is hot, add the prawns and cook until lightly golden on the outside and slightly raw in the centres, 40 to 50 seconds on each side. Season with salt and pepper and set aside.

Heat another pan over medium heat and add 1 tbsp of the ghee. When the ghee is hot, add the mushrooms and cook until tender, 2 minutes. Add the spring onion, bean sprouts, and tamari. Stir in the prawns and reserved vegetables and cook for 1 minute; set aside.

To make the omelette, heat a 10-inch non-stick frying pan over medium heat and add the remaining 1 tsp ghee. When the ghee is hot, add the egg mixture to the pan and swirl the pan to coat the bottom of the pan with the eggs. Cook just until the egg mixture is lightly golden underneath and moist on the top, 40 to 60 seconds. Slide the omelette out of the pan and onto a cutting board. Spoon the prawn-vegetable filling onto the centre of the omelette in a line. Roll up the omelette and cut in half to form two rolls. Place a rolled omelette, cut side up, in each of two serving bowls and ladle over the broth. Sprinkle with bonito flakes, black sesame seeds, and drizzle with sesame oil. Garnish with spring onions and microgreens, if using, and serve.

Liquorice root is a wonderful ingredient with remarkable healing properties and a uniquely sweet flavour. I often pop liquorice root into my smoothies, stocks, braises, burgers, and meatballs to add natural sweetness. I've made these sausages into patties so that the eggs have nice beds to sit upon. This way, when you crack the egg yolk, it mixes in with the meat and creates a yummy sauce that is divine with the meat and greens. Feel free to add sautéed mushrooms or broccoli to this dish and serve it for breakfast, lunch, or dinner. If you can't get hold of any liquorice root, just leave it out or add some cumin instead.

LIQUORICE ROOT SAUSAGES
WITH FRIED EGGS & GREENS

SERVES 4

1 tbsp ground liquorice root or ground cumin

½ tsp whole cloves

¼ tsp coriander seeds

¼ tsp white pepper

1¼ lb (550 g) minced pork

2 cloves garlic, finely chopped

4 sprigs thyme, finely chopped

1 tbsp chopped fresh parsley

4 tbsp beef tallow, duck fat, coconut oil, or ghee

½ bunch of Swiss chard, stems removed and leaves torn

4 eggs

¼ bunch of chives, finely chopped

Chilli oil

In a spice grinder or using a mortar and pestle, grind together the liquorice root, cloves, coriander, white pepper, and 1 tsp sea salt to make a fine powder. Transfer the spice mix to a bowl and stir in 2 tbsp cold water. Add the pork, garlic, thyme, and parsley and mix by hand to combine. Refrigerate for 20 minutes to allow the flavours to infuse the mixture.

Divide the meat mixture into four portions and form into patties about 3 inches (8 cm) in diameter and ¾ inch (2 cm) thick.

Heat a large non-stick frying pan over medium heat and add 2 tbsp of the beef tallow. When the tallow is melted and hot, add the patties and cook for about 3 minutes per side, or until cooked through and golden. Keep warm.

Meanwhile, heat another non-stick frying pan over medium heat and add 1 tbsp beef tallow. When the fat melts, add the Swiss chard and sauté until just wilted, 2 minutes. Season with salt and freshly cracked black pepper. Remove from the pan and set aside; keep warm.

Wipe the frying pan clean and return to the stove over medium-low heat. Add the remaining 1 tbsp beef tallow. When the fat is melted and hot, carefully crack the eggs into the frying pan and cook, undisturbed, until the whites are cooked through and the yolks are still runny, 2 to 3 minutes, or until cooked to your liking.

To serve, divide the Swiss chard between four serving plates; top each portion with a sausage patty and fried egg. To finish, sprinkle over some chopped chives, drizzle with chilli oil, and season with salt and pepper.

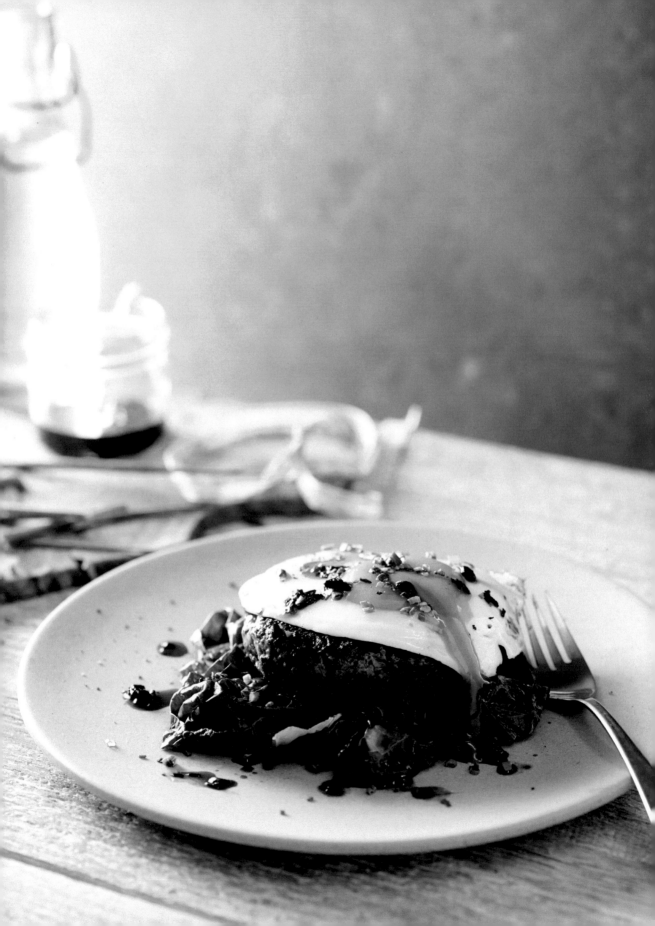

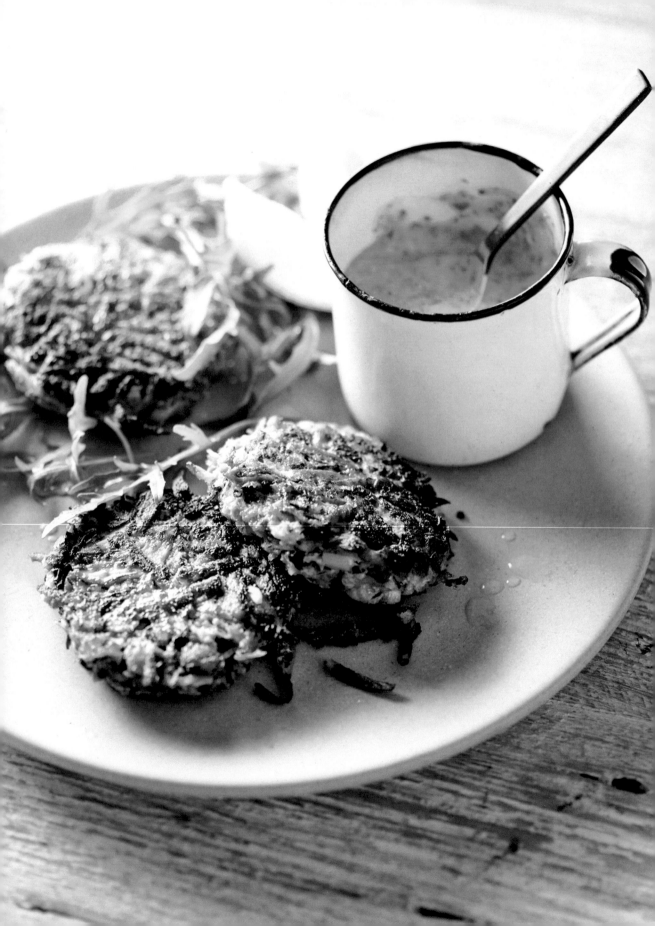

Courgettes are wonderful to work with. Full of vitamin C and other phytonutrients, they are at their peak in the warmer summer months. A great way to introduce courgettes into your kid's diet is to make these courgette fritters. The fritters become even more delicious when you serve them with a variety of dressings. My partner Nic loves to dip hers into green goddess dressing (page 204); my eldest daughter, Chilli, loves to dip her fritters into green tahini (tahini with chopped coriander); and my youngest daughter, Indii, loves to dip hers into homemade harissa (page 205). I love them with a simple squeeze of lemon juice and a sprinkling of dried red chilli flakes.

COURGETTE & FENNEL FRITTERS

SERVES 4 TO 6

17½ oz (500 g) courgettes, grated

9 oz (250 g) sweet potato or carrots, peeled and grated

1¾ oz (50 g) fennel bulb, shaved

2 tbsp chopped fresh flat-leaf parsley leaves

2 tbsp chopped fresh mint leaves

4 spring onions, sliced

Finely grated zest of 1 lemon

3 eggs

½ cup (50 g) ground almonds, plus more as needed

4 tbsp ghee or coconut oil, for cooking

to serve

1 cup (250 ml) green goddess dressing (page 204)

About 2 handfuls of rocket

Lemon wedges

Combine the courgette and sweet potato in a colander. Sprinkle with a good pinch of sea salt and mix through. Let sit for 15 minutes.

Squeeze out all the moisture from the courgette and sweet potato with your hands; I like to grab handfuls and squeeze out as much liquid as I can. You can also wrap it in a clean tea towel and squeeze the liquid out. Put the grated courgette, sweet potato, and fennel into a large bowl. Add the parsley, mint, spring onions, lemon zest, eggs, ground almonds, and a few grinds of cracked black pepper. Mix well until incorporated. At this stage it's good to test and cook a fritter to make sure it holds together well. Add a touch more ground almonds, if needed. Form into small patties about 2½ inches (6 cm) in diameter.

Heat a frying pan over medium heat and add the ghee. When the ghee is hot, add the fritters and cook until golden, turning once, about 4 minutes. Serve with the green goddess dressing, rocket, and lemon wedges.

On my first overseas surfing holiday, I traveled to the island of Bali. The first thing I noticed when I hopped off the plane was the distinct smell: a combination of odours from the land and sea that created a kind of sautéed Asian bouquet, primarily because it's so flipping hot. As you can imagine, my chef instincts were attracted to the busy food stalls and restaurants, where the first local delicacy I ate was one of Bali's national treasures, *nasi goreng*, which translates as fried rice. It's flavoured with garlic, tamarind, and chillies, then served with egg plus chicken, dried fish, or prawns. Here's my Paleo-inspired version, using cauliflower instead of rice.

NASI GORENG

SERVES 4

4 tbsp coconut oil

14 oz (400 g) boneless, skinless chicken thighs, cut into ½-inch (2 cm) pieces

5 oz (150 g) bacon rashers, thinly sliced crosswise

4 shallots, thinly sliced

2 cloves garlic, finely chopped

1 carrot, peeled and finely diced

1 celery stalk, trimmed and finely diced

1 fresh red chilli, seeded and finely chopped

5 oz (150 g) cooked, peeled prawns

½ cup (50 g) finely shredded Chinese cabbage

1 tsp prawn paste

3 cups (600 g) Cauliflower Rice (page 61)

1 cup (120 g) bean sprouts

2 spring onions, sliced

2 tbsp fried shallots (page 207)

3 tbsp wheat-free tamari or coconut aminos

1 tbsp fish sauce

1 tsp tamarind pulp

4 eggs

Bird's eye chillies, thinly sliced

Lime wedges

Place a large wok over medium heat, add 2 tbsp of the coconut oil, and heat until just smoking. Add half the chicken and stir-fry until brown and just cooked through, 3 minutes. Transfer to a bowl, then stir-fry the remaining chicken and transfer to the bowl. Add the bacon to the wok and stir-fry until it becomes golden and crispy, 2 minutes. Transfer to the bowl with the chicken and set aside.

Add 1 tbsp coconut oil to the wok and heat over medium heat. Add the shallots and garlic and stir-fry until shallots are soft, 1 minute. Add the carrot, celery, and red chilli and stir-fry for 3 minutes.

Return the cooked chicken and bacon to the wok, add the prawns and cabbage, and stir-fry until the cabbage wilts, 3 minutes. Stir in the prawn paste, then add the cauliflower rice, bean sprouts, spring onions, 1 tbsp of the fried shallots, the tamari, fish sauce, and tamarind pulp. Stir-fry until heated through, 2 minutes. Transfer to a large bowl and cover with foil to keep warm.

Heat the remaining 1 tbsp coconut oil in a large non-stick frying pan over medium-high heat. When hot, crack the eggs into the pan and cook, uncovered, until the whites set and the yolks are almost set (for a soft yolk), 2 minutes, or until cooked to your liking. Transfer to a plate.

Spoon the *nasi goreng* into four shallow serving bowls. Top each with a fried egg and sprinkle over the remaining 1 tbsp fried shallots. Serve, accompanied by chilli slices and lime wedges.

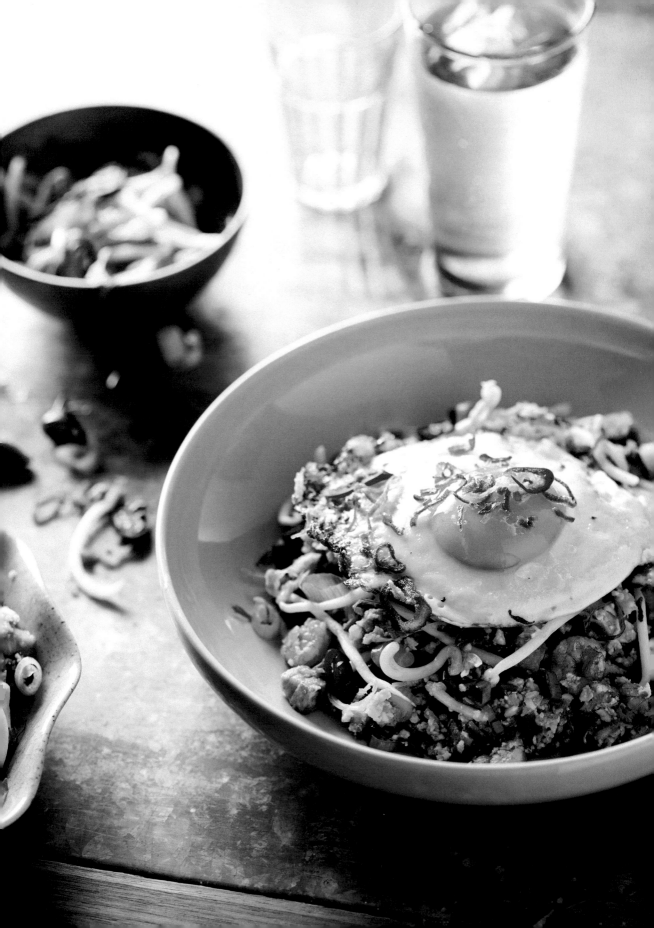

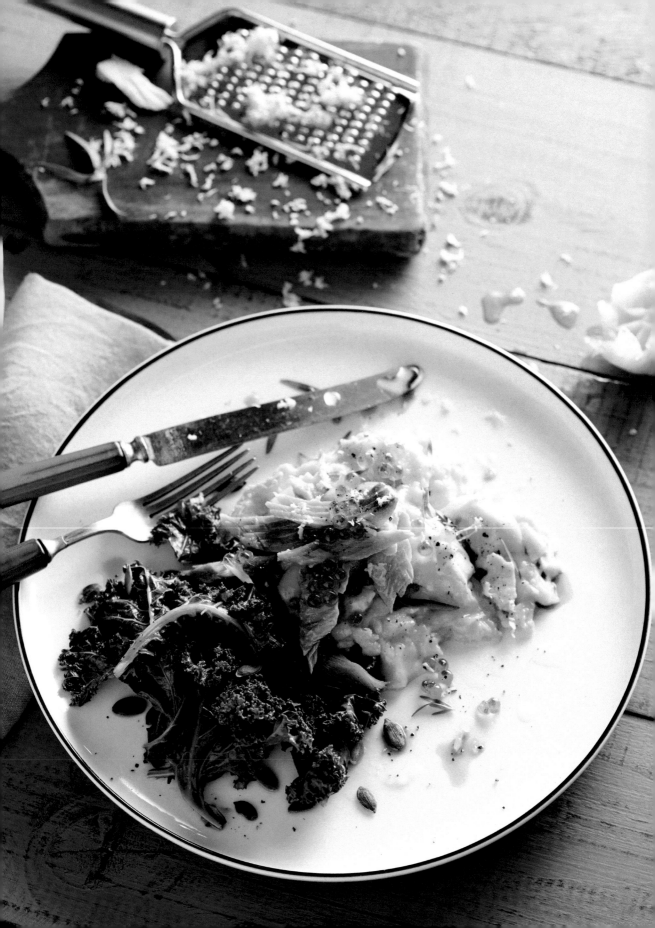

Often overlooked in the grocery store or the farmers' market, horseradish can enhance the most humble of ingredients and turn them into something rather sublime. One of my favourite ways to complement protein is with a light sprinkling of freshly grated horseradish. It also works well as a final touch to a slow-braised dish to give it some excitement, or mixed into Steak Tartare (page 143). It is particularly good with seafood. For this recipe, I've married fresh horseradish with mouth-watering smoked trout and creamy scrambled eggs to create a delectable partnership of flavour.

SCRAMBLED EGGS
WITH SMOKED TROUT, KALE & HORSERADISH
SERVES 2

4 eggs

2 tbsp coconut cream

8 fresh tarragon leaves, torn

2 tbsp ghee or coconut oil

¼ bunch of kale, stems removed, leaves torn

3½ tbsp (30 g) pumpkin seeds

8½ oz (240 g) smoked trout, flaked

2 tbsp (30 g) trout roe or salmon roe

Freshly grated horseradish

Lemon wedges

Whisk together the eggs, coconut cream, half the tarragon, a pinch of sea salt, and some freshly cracked black pepper in a bowl.

In a non-stick frying pan over medium heat, heat 1 tbsp of the ghee until hot. Pour in the egg mixture and stir gently with a wooden spoon until the eggs are set, 2 to 3 minutes.

Meanwhile, in another frying pan, heat the remaining 1 tbsp of ghee over medium-high heat. Add the kale and pumpkin seeds and sauté until the kale is tender and wilted, 3 to 5 minutes; season with salt and pepper.

Divide the kale between two plates. Top the kale with the eggs, then top the eggs with the trout. Finish with salmon roe, grated horseradish, and the remaining tarragon. Serve with lemon wedges.

Chia seeds come from a flowering plant in the mint family that's native to Mexico and Guatemala. History suggests that chia seeds were an important food crop for the Aztecs. The little seed, which can be white, dark brown, or black in colour, also has a substantial nutritional profile. Chia seeds contain calcium, manganese, and phosphorus and are a great source of protein and healthy omega-3 fats. One of my favourite ways to enjoy the seeds is in these gorgeous little puddings that my partner, Nic, makes once a week. If you can't find a fresh young coconut, use packaged coconut water and omit the flesh, or use more coconut milk or cream and adjust the amount of honey to taste. You will still make an amazing dish!

BLACK CHIA SEED PUDDINGS
WITH NUTS, FIGS & DATES

SERVES 2

1 young green coconut

½ cup (125 ml) coconut cream

½ cup (50 g) black chia seeds

1 to 2 tbsp raw honey or a tiny pinch green leaf stevia powder

⅓ cup (50 g) Brazil nuts, activated (page 209) and chopped

⅓ cup (45 g) macadamia nuts, activated (page 209) and chopped

4 fresh figs, cut into wedges

4 fresh medjool dates, pitted and sliced

Open the top of the coconut and pour out the coconut water into a measuring cup. Remove the coconut flesh out of the shell and roughly chop. Combine it with ½ cup (125 ml) of the coconut water in a food processor. Whirl it in the food processor until you have a smooth, thick puree. (If you have any remaining coconut water, drink it straight away or store it in the refrigerator for up to a week.)

In a bowl, combine the coconut puree, coconut cream, chia seeds, and honey and mix well to combine. Transfer the mixture to two glasses and refrigerate for at least 2 hours before serving, until set. (You can make these up to 2 days in advance, if you like.)

Remove the pudding from the refrigerator and garnish with the nuts, figs, and dates. Drizzle with a little more honey, if desired.

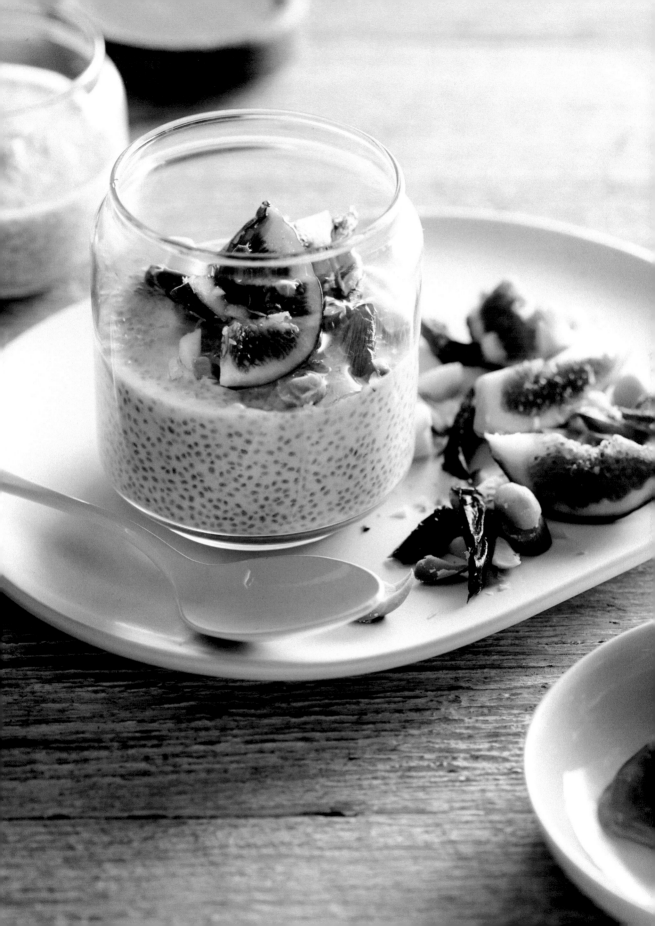

VEGETABLES, SIDES & SNACKS

42
sweet potato fries with
rosemary & sage

45
kale chips with garlic
& sun-dried tomato

46
kale hummus

49
nori chips with sesame

50
raw cauliflower tabbouleh

53
moroccan carrot salad

54
chopped salad

57
warm baby beetroot &
sorrel salad with cashew
cheese & walnuts

58
root vegetable slaw with
chervil mayonnaise

61
cauliflower rice

62
sautéed greens with
lemon & garlic

65
water spinach with
garlic & chillies

66
sauerkraut with
carrots & apples

69
brussels sprouts with
bacon & garlic

70
raw courgette lasagna with
tomato-olive pesto

73
roasted winter vegetables

Sweet potato fries are a must-have side for certain dishes, and even though we limit the amount of starch we consume, we still enjoy these on our monthly fish and chips night. They're sublime when dipped in some homemade harissa, aïoli, or pesto. This recipe is also delicious if you're serving them with a roast because you can season all the other veggies with the same herbs.

SWEET POTATO FRIES
WITH ROSEMARY & SAGE

SERVES 4 TO 6

4 tbsp coconut oil, melted, plus more for the baking sheet

1¾ lb (800 g) sweet potatoes, peeled and cut into ¼-inch (6 mm) slices, then cut into ¼-inch (6 mm) strips

3 sprigs rosemary, coarsely chopped

10 fresh sage leaves, coarsely chopped

Chipotle aïoli (page 203), for serving

Preheat the oven to 400°F (200°C gas 6). Lightly coat a large baking sheet with coconut oil.

Combine the coconut oil, sweet potatoes, rosemary, sage, ½ tsp sea salt, and ½ tsp freshly cracked black pepper in a large bowl. Toss to coat. Spread the fries on the baking sheet in a single layer so they are not touching one another.

Bake for 10 minutes. Turn the fries over. Continue baking for about 5 minutes more, until the fries are tender and lightly browned. Serve right away with the chipotle aïoli.

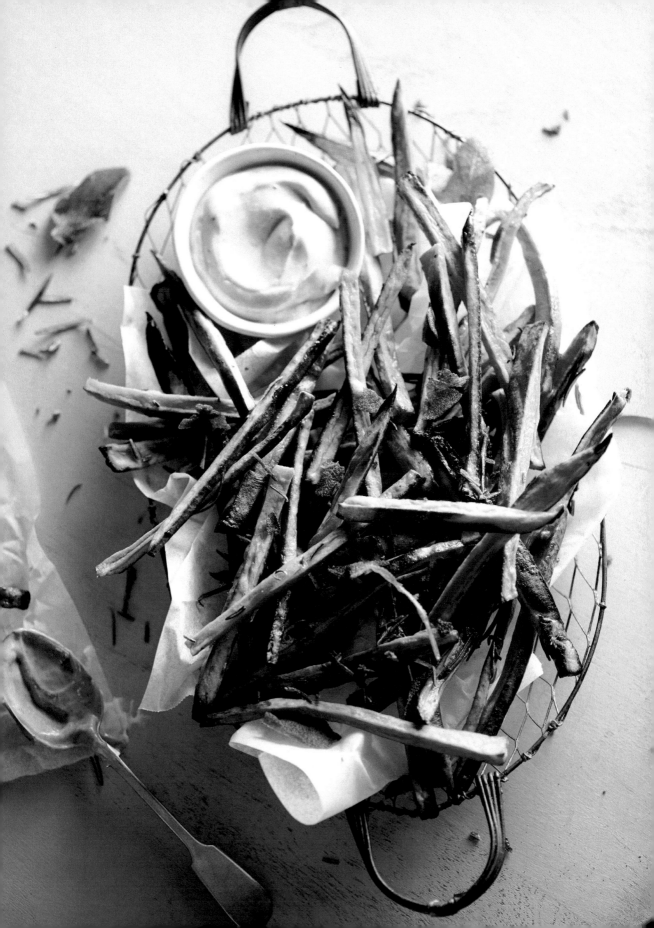

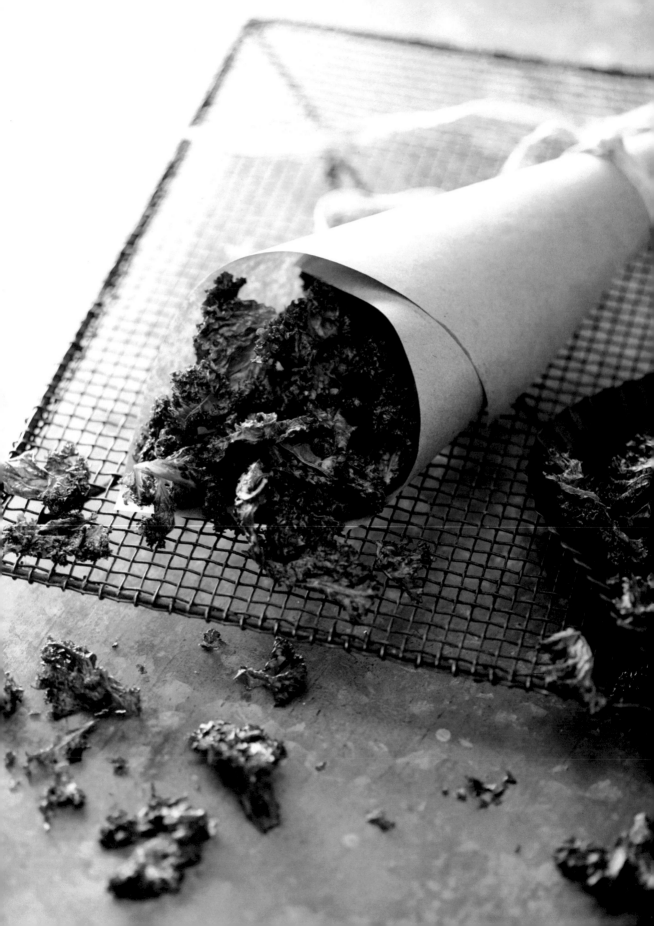

These chips are remarkably moreish, so be prepared to bake countless batches! My partner, Nic, makes this crispy green goodness almost daily because they disappear as soon as they come out of the oven. The beauty of kale chips is that you can flavour them in so many different ways with spices, herbs, nuts, seeds, and veggies. Serve them on their own as a snack, toss them into salads, sprinkle them on slow-roasted veggies, or even add them as a finishing touch to canapés, such as Tuna Tartare on Nori Crisps (page 81). For something exciting, toss the kale chips with grated dehydrated carrot, ground cumin and coriander, and cashews.

KALE CHIPS
WITH GARLIC & SUN-DRIED TOMATO
SERVES 2 TO 4

⅓ cup (40 g) sunflower seeds, activated (page 209) then soaked overnight

2¾ oz (80 g) oil-packed sun-dried tomatoes, drained and patted dry

1 clove garlic, peeled

2 tbsp freshly squeezed lemon juice

3 tbsp coconut oil, plus more for greasing

1 large bunch of kale, tough stems removed, leaves torn into large pieces (about 10 oz/300 g)

Combine the sunflower seeds, sun-dried tomatoes, garlic clove, lemon juice, coconut oil, and ¼ tsp sea salt in a food processor and blend to make a slightly coarse paste. Transfer the paste to a large bowl, add the kale, and toss to coat evenly. Season with more salt if you like.

Preheat the oven to 250°F (120°C gas ½). Grease a large baking sheet with coconut oil and line with baking parchment.

Arrange the kale in a single layer on the prepared baking sheet and bake for 40 to 50 minutes, or until crispy. Start checking after 30 minutes; don't overcook or they'll burn! Remove from the oven and cool.

Kale is full of antioxidants; iron; vitamins A, C, and K; and calcium. It is also a great detox food and a powerful anti-inflammatory. In other words, kale has a lot going for it. This recipe for kale hummus is a favourite in our house. We even put it in the kids' lunch boxes along with some fresh vegetables (like sliced carrots, radishes, cucumber, and celery) for dipping. Instead of the kale, you can use spinach or beetroot leaves, or a combination, if you like.

KALE HUMMUS

SERVES 6

1 tbsp coconut oil

1 onion, diced

4 cloves garlic, finely chopped

1 bunch of kale, stemmed and chopped

½ cup (125 ml) chicken stock (page 202) or water

½ cup (120 g) unhulled tahini

3 tbsp extra virgin olive oil, plus more if needed

2 tbsp freshly squeezed lemon juice

4 tbsp macadamia nuts, activated (page 209)

Pinch of cayenne pepper

Cut fresh vegetables, such as carrots, radishes, and fennel, to serve

In a large saucepan over medium heat, heat the coconut oil until melted and hot. Add the onion and cook, stirring, until softened, about 5 minutes. Add the garlic and cook for about 30 seconds, or until it starts to colour. Add the kale and the chicken stock. Cover and cook until the kale is tender, about 3 minutes.

Transfer the kale mixture and the cooking liquid to a food processor and let cool for a few minutes. Add the tahini, olive oil, lemon juice, macadamia nuts, cayenne, and sea salt and freshly cracked black pepper to taste. Process until smooth. Add a little more oil if needed. Transfer to a bowl and serve with vegetables alongside for dipping.

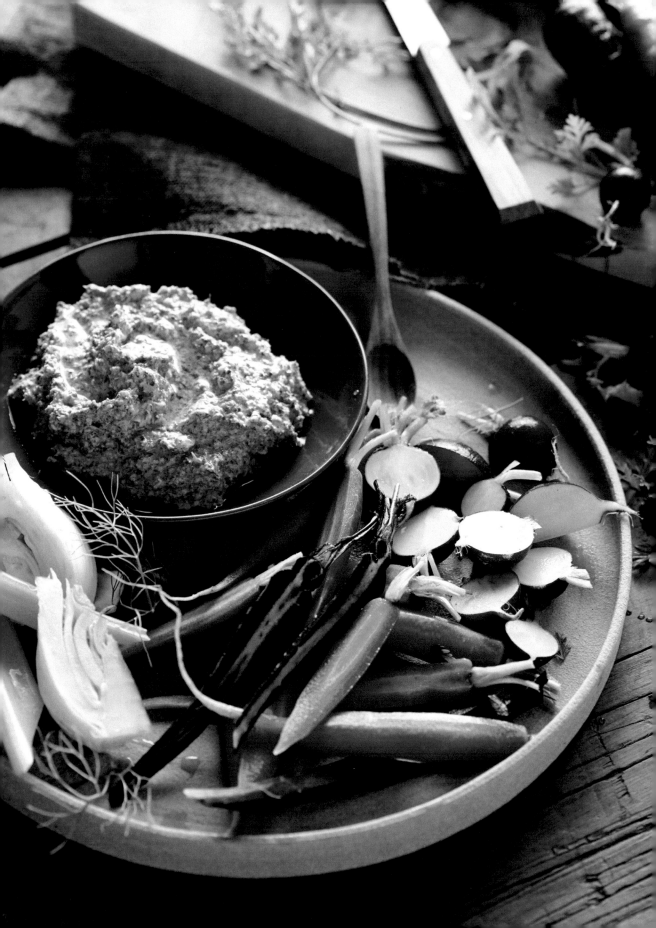

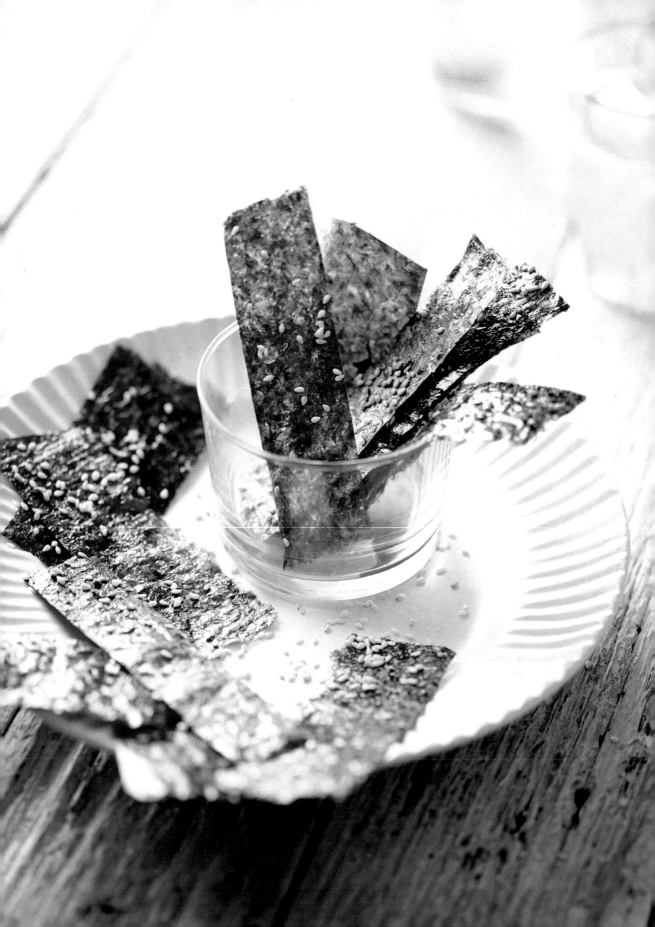

I live with three girls who also like to be known as mermaids, so they love to munch on nosh from the sea, especially anything with seaweed, whether it be wakame in their miso; a kombu, hijiki, and daikon salad; or just plain nori sheets on their own. So, every once in a while, I spoil my mermaids with this popular Japanese treat, which is simple, quick, healthy, and delicious!

NORI CHIPS
WITH SESAME
SERVES 4

1 tbsp sesame seeds

1 tbsp toasted sesame oil or melted coconut oil

8 sheets nori

Preheat the oven to 350° (180°C gas 4).

Using a pestle and mortar, grind the sesame seeds and ½ tsp sea salt to a coarse powder. Dip a pastry brush in the sesame oil and brush the nori sheets with sesame oil, covering the whole sheet with the oil. Place the oiled nori sheets on baking sheets, without overlapping the nori sheets. Place in the oven to toast until crisp, 4 to 5 minutes. Remove from the oven and while hot, sprinkle with the sesame salt. Cut into squares and store in an airtight container for up to 3 months.

Tabbouleh is a favourite Middle Eastern salad containing tomatoes, cucumbers, fresh herbs such as parsley and mint, garlic, lemon juice, salt, olive oil, and usually bulgur or couscous, which are both made from wheat. With this recipe, I have replaced the wheat with toasted sesame seeds and very finely chopped cauliflower to add texture, and, more importantly, flavour. I have also added some very thinly sliced okra. Okra is full of amazing health benefits. When it is in season, it features in a multitude of dishes on our family table, from raw preparations like this one to curries, stir-fries, and soups.

RAW CAULIFLOWER TABBOULEH
SERVES 4 TO 6

½ head cauliflower, cut into large chunks

½ cup (125 ml) freshly squeezed lemon juice

⅓ cup (80 ml) extra virgin olive oil

1 clove garlic, finely chopped

2 tsp ground sumac, plus more to serve

1 tsp ground cumin

1 cup (60 g) chopped fresh flat-leaf parsley

½ cup (30 g) packed chopped fresh mint

1 large fennel bulb, finely diced

1 red onion, finely chopped

2 cucumbers, preferably Lebanese, chopped

8 okra pods, sliced crosswise

1 carrot, peeled and shredded

8 oz (200 g) tomatoes, chopped into large dice

1 tbsp white sesame seeds, toasted

In a food processor, process the cauliflower until it resembles coarse grains. To make the dressing, whisk together the lemon juice, olive oil, garlic, sumac, and cumin and set aside.

In a large serving bowl, combine the cauliflower with the parsley, mint, fennel, red onion, cucumbers, okra, carrot, and tomatoes. Mix in the dressing, season with sea salt and freshly cracked black pepper, and let marinate for 10 minutes.

To serve, sprinkle with toasted sesame seeds and a little sumac. Serve at once.

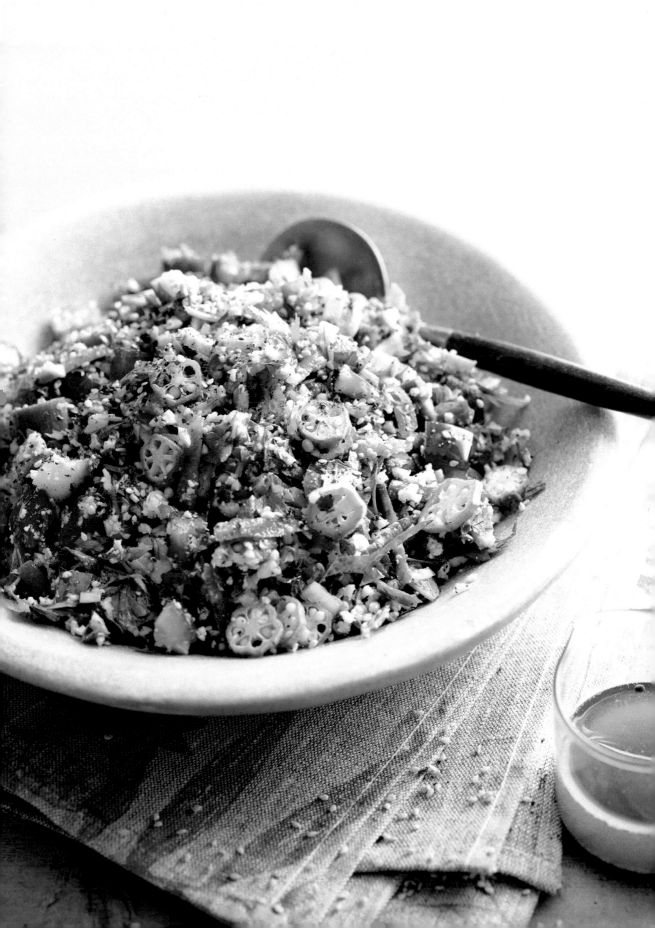

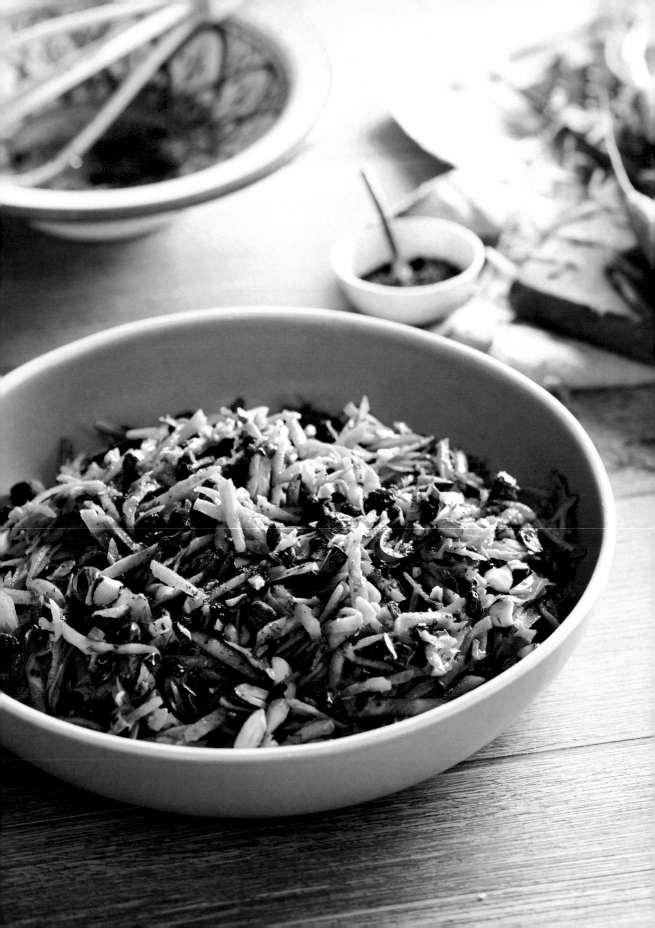

I'm a big fan of Moroccan cuisine because it uses harmonious blends of herbs and spices to create flavours that will tantalize even the most judicious taste buds. This carrot salad is a knockout when served with many different dishes, but especially lamb, roasted chicken, or spiced fish. It's a great one to keep in the fridge, too. It is terrific to serve on a piece of sprouted bread with some sliced avocado and liver pâté to really top it off.

MOROCCAN CARROT SALAD

SERVES 4

⅓ cup (80 ml) extra virgin olive oil

1 tbsp freshly squeezed lemon juice

1 tbsp raw apple cider vinegar

1 tbsp raw honey

1 tsp peeled and grated fresh ginger

1 fresh red chilli, seeded and finely chopped

½ tsp ground sumac

4 large carrots, peeled and grated

Handful of almonds activated (page 209), toasted, and chopped

Large handful of chopped fresh coriander

Handful of fresh mint leaves, chopped

¼ cup (40 g) dried barberries or currants

In a large serving bowl, whisk together the olive oil, lemon juice, vinegar, honey, and ginger until well combined. Add the chilli, sumac, carrots, almonds, coriander, mint, and barberries or currants. Toss, season with sea salt and freshly cracked black pepper, and serve.

Salads are something that I look forward to eating every day, so I often chop up enough ingredients for a few meals. If you do this, too, be sure to only dress the amount you want to consume in one meal so the dressing doesn't make the rest of the salad soggy. When serving salads, I like to put out bowls of activated nuts and seeds, which add texture and good fats to the meal, as well as bowls of fresh herbs (if they aren't already in the salad), so everyone can sprinkle on what they like. Here is a recipe for a simple chopped salad that you can play around with, using whatever's in season.

CHOPPED SALAD

SERVES 4 TO 6

dressing
2 tbsp raw apple cider vinegar or sherry vinegar

1 tbsp freshly squeezed lemon juice

1 tsp fermented mustard (page 206)

⅓ cup (80 ml) good-quality extra virgin olive oil

salad
3 vine-ripened tomatoes, seeded and diced

2 cucumbers, Lebanese type preferred, diced

1 head baby cos lettuce, chopped

1 cup (80 g) shredded red cabbage

1 red pepper, seeded and diced

1 fresh red chilli, seeded and finely chopped

2 shallots, sliced

2 tbsp chopped fresh flat-leaf parsley

2 tbsp chopped fresh coriander

1 tbsp chopped fresh mint leaves

1 avocado, halved, pitted, peeled, and diced

⅓ cup (40 g) pumpkin seeds, activated (page 209)

¼ cup (30 g) sunflower seeds, activated (page 209)

To make the dressing, combine the vinegar, lemon juice, and mustard in a bowl and whisk to combine. Slowly add the olive oil in a slow steady stream until incorporated through. Season with sea salt and freshly cracked black pepper.

To make the salad, combine the tomatoes, cucumbers, lettuce, red cabbage, red pepper, chilli, shallots, parsley, coriander, mint, avocado, pumpkin seeds, and sunflower seeds in a bowl. Add the dressing and toss. Season with salt and pepper to taste. Allow the salad to stand for 10 minutes to marinate before serving.

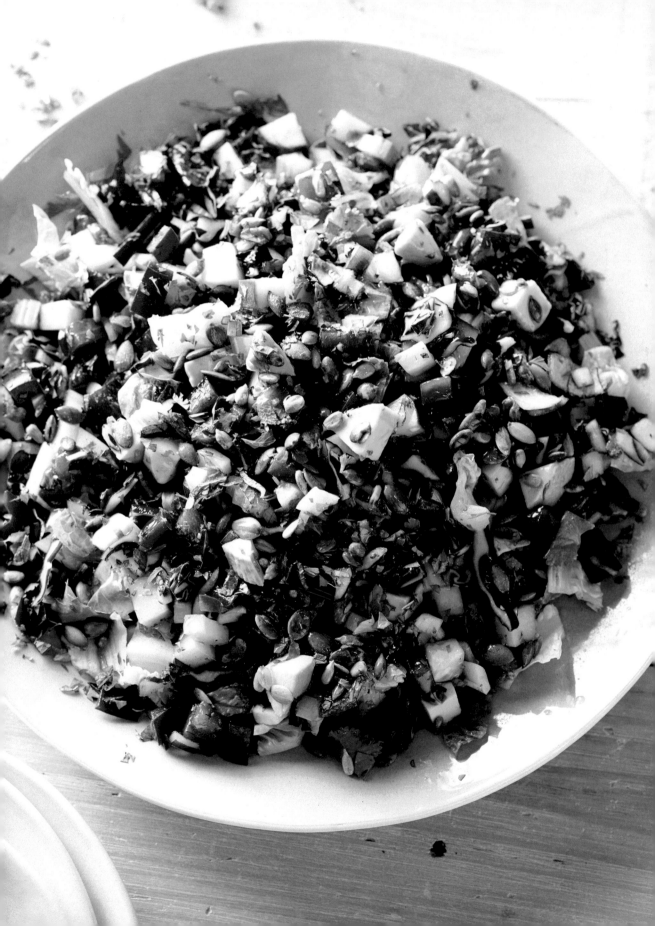

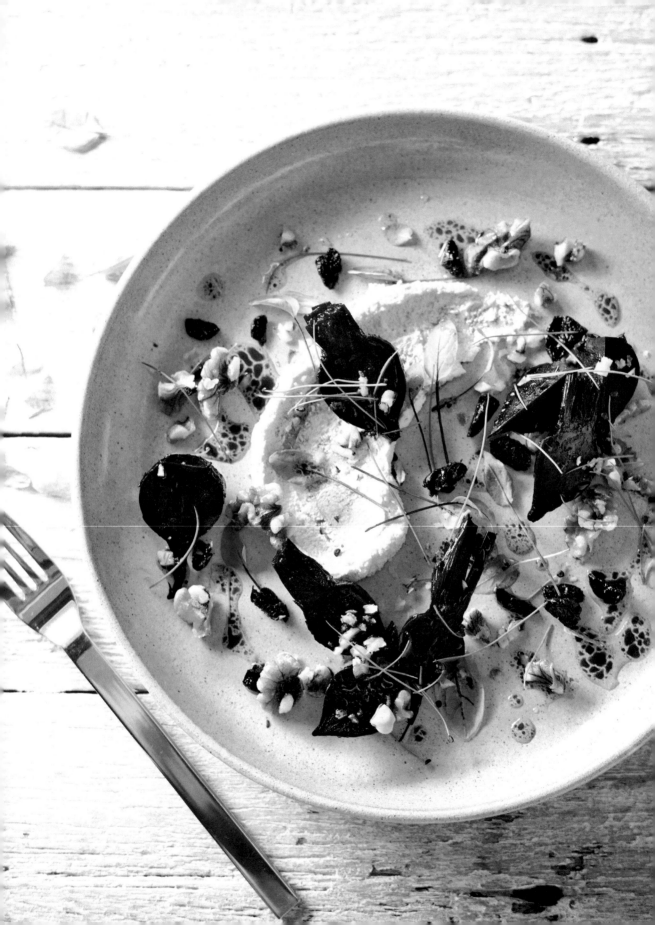

You have to love beetroots for being so outrageous in their colour, whether they are the standard purple or the ever-increasing golden varieties seen at farmers' markets. Did you know that beetroots were used as an aphrodisiac during Roman times? Turns out beetroots contain high amounts of boron, which directly relates to the production of human sex hormones. If that little tidbit of information, plus the fact that beetroots are nutritional powerhouses, isn't enough to get you popping them onto the menu on a weekly basis, then perhaps this recipe will help. Beetroots are renowned for partnering beautifully with cheese, especially goat cheese, and they are often paired with nuts, so I thought the addition of nut cheese would work here, and it does – splendidly.

WARM BABY BEETROOT & SORREL SALAD
WITH CASHEW CHEESE & WALNUTS
SERVES 4

2 bunches of baby red beetroots (about 20), trimmed and halved, or quartered if large

Coconut oil, melted, for drizzling

⅓ cup (80 ml) extra virgin olive oil

2 tbsp good-quality red wine or apple cider vinegar

2 tsp freshly squeezed lemon juice

1 cup (100 g) walnuts, activated (page 209), toasted, and coarsely chopped

1 cup (200 g) cashew or macadamia cheese (page 208)

½ bunch of chives, cut into 2-inch (5 cm) lengths

1 handful of sorrel leaves, red-veined preferred

½ cup packed (80 g) dried cherries, coarsely chopped

On a large piece of aluminium foil, toss the beetroots with a little melted coconut oil until lightly coated. Wrap the foil around the beetroots and seal. Place on a baking sheet and roast for 40 minutes, or until tender. When the beetroots are cool enough to touch, peel off the skins.

Combine the olive oil, red wine vinegar, lemon juice, and half of the walnuts in a screw-top jar with a little sea salt and freshly cracked black pepper. Shake well.

Thickly spread the cashew cheese on a large platter and top with the warm beetroots. Drizzle the beetroots with some of the dressing, and then scatter over the chives, sorrel, and dried cherries. Season with salt and pepper. Garnish with the remaining walnuts. Serve warm. Pass the remaining dressing at the table.

The raw food movement has really taken off, and research shows that adopting an all plant-based diet can be beneficial for a period of time to cleanse the body. I like to eat a portion of my food raw – including vegetables, meat, and seafood – as I find it makes me feel great. This raw, crunchy salad is an excellent dish to add to your repertoire alongside pretty much any meal featured in this book. It's a great way of getting some beneficial micronutrients into your body.

ROOT VEGETABLE SLAW
WITH CHERVIL MAYONNAISE

SERVES 4 TO 6

2 beetroots, peeled

2 carrots, peeled

½ celeriac, peeled

1 kohlrabi bulb, peeled

¼ head red cabbage, cored and shredded

1 large handful of thinly sliced fennel bulb

½ cup (120 ml) aïoli (page 203)

Juice of 1 lemon

3 tbsp chopped fresh chervil

2 large handfuls of fresh mint leaves, shredded

2 handfuls of fresh flat-leaf parsley leaves, coarsely chopped

½ tbsp finely grated lemon zest

Slice the beetroots, carrots, celeriac, and kohlrabi paper thin. Stack a few slices at a time on top of each other and cut them into matchstick strips. Alternatively, use a mandoline or a food processor with the appropriate attachment. Combine all the strips, the cabbage, and fennel in a large bowl and cover with cold water. Set aside.

To make the chervil mayonnaise, combine the aïoli, lemon juice, and chervil and mix well.

Drain the vegetables and dry well with paper towels. Dry the bowl and return the vegetables to the bowl.

When you are ready to serve, add the mint, parsley, lemon zest, 1 tsp freshly cracked black pepper, and chervil mayonnaise. Toss well, taste, and add sea salt if needed. Serve at once.

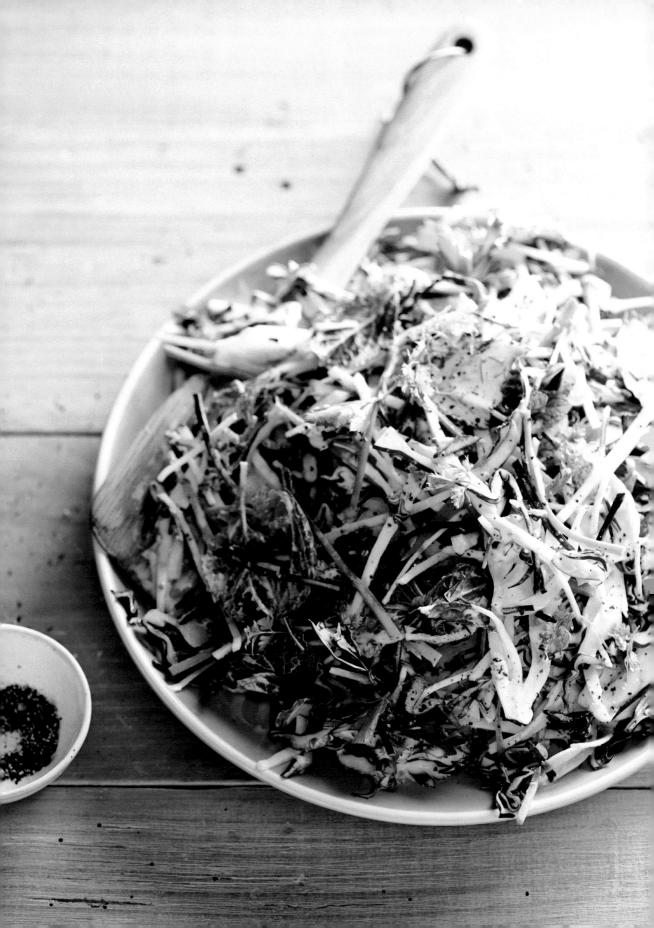

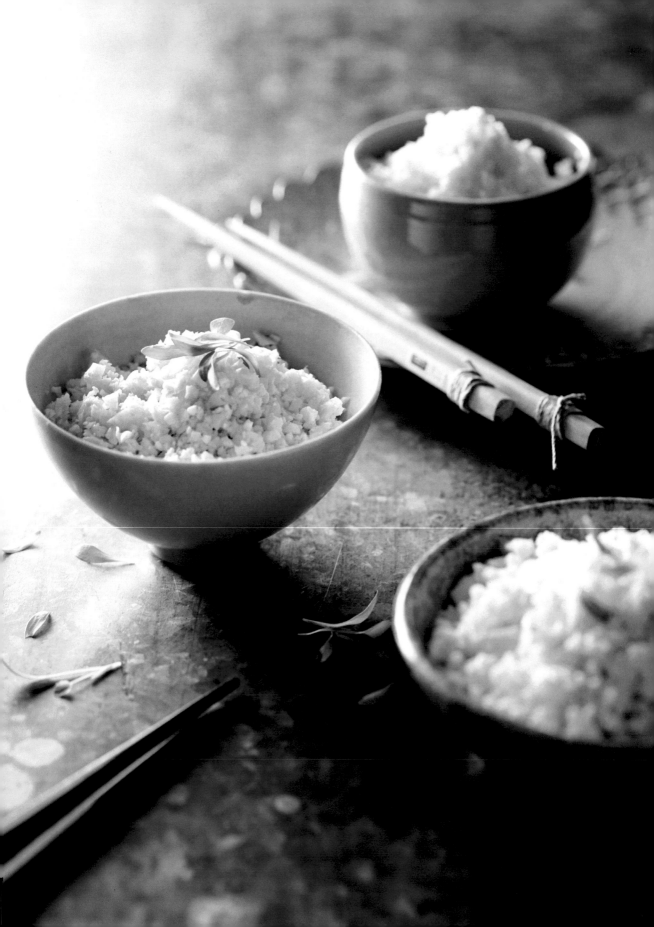

The Paleo diet eliminates grains so that our bodies have the opportunity to find a healthy balance in weight, energy levels, and general well-being. Rice was the hardest grain for me to eliminate from my diet because I was addicted to eating sushi and rice with curry. So I faced a small problem: if I was going to embrace the Paleo lifestyle wholeheartedly, I needed to find an alternative to rice. The answer for me is this cauliflower rice. It works well with curries, braises, even as a substitute for sushi rice (you just need to bind it with avocado and a little tahini).

CAULIFLOWER RICE

SERVES 4

1 head cauliflower, chopped   2 tbsp coconut oil   Chopped fresh coriander or other herbs, to garnish

Put the cauliflower in a food processor and pulse into tiny, fine pieces that look like grains of rice.

Heat the coconut oil in a frying pan over medium heat. Add the cauliflower and lightly cook until softened, 3 to 4 minutes. Season with sea salt and freshly cracked black pepper. Garnish with coriander and serve.

A big bowl of green vegetables on the table is one of the key ingredients I rely upon to build and maintain my health, so I am going to keep this introduction short and sweet, which is, incidentally, how long it takes to whip up this appetizing dish. I can't encourage this enough: 'Please eat your greens!' I include green beans here because I think they are more pod than bean, but feel free to replace them with okra.

SAUTÉED GREENS
WITH LEMON & GARLIC
SERVES 4

1 bunch of green asparagus

1 bunch of broccolini, trimmed and halved

¼ cup (50 g) coconut oil, beef tallow, duck fat, or ghee

2 cloves garlic, sliced

2 courgettes, thinly sliced

5 oz (150 g) fresh green beans, okra, or asparagus

½ bunch of kale, tough stems removed and leaves coarsely chopped

Finely grated zest and juice of 1 lemon

Bring a large pan of water to a boil. Add the asparagus and broccolini and blanch just until tender, 2 to 3 minutes. Plunge into an ice bath or very cold water to stop the cooking.

Meanwhile, heat the oil in a large frying pan over medium heat, add the garlic, and cook until it is fragrant, about 1 minute. Just before the garlic starts to colour, add the courgettes and cook until slightly golden, about 30 seconds. Add the asparagus, broccolini, green beans, and kale and sauté until the broccolini becomes crisp, 2 minutes. Add the lemon zest and juice, season with sea salt and freshly cracked black pepper, and serve.

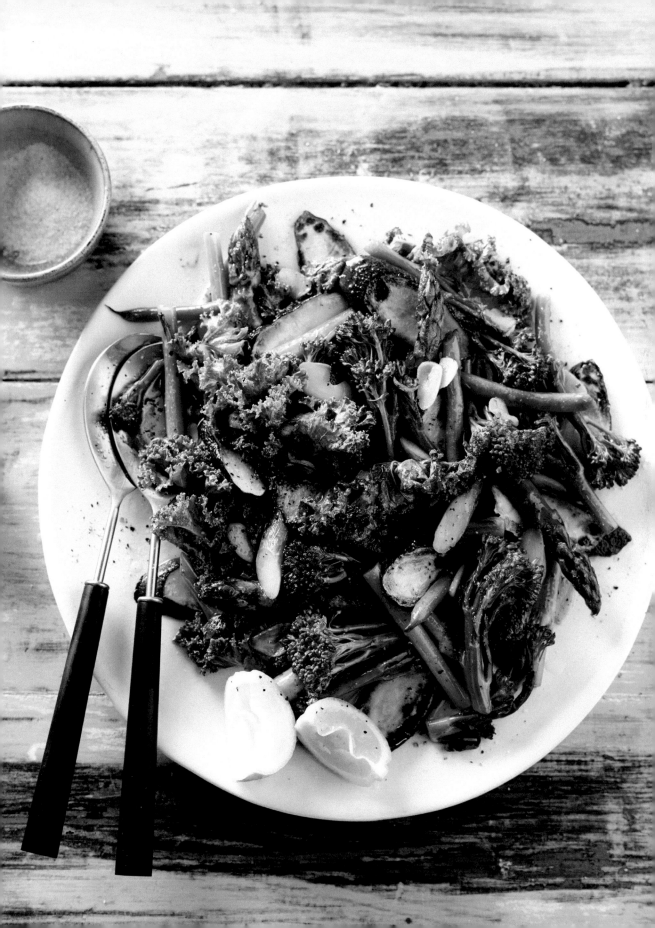

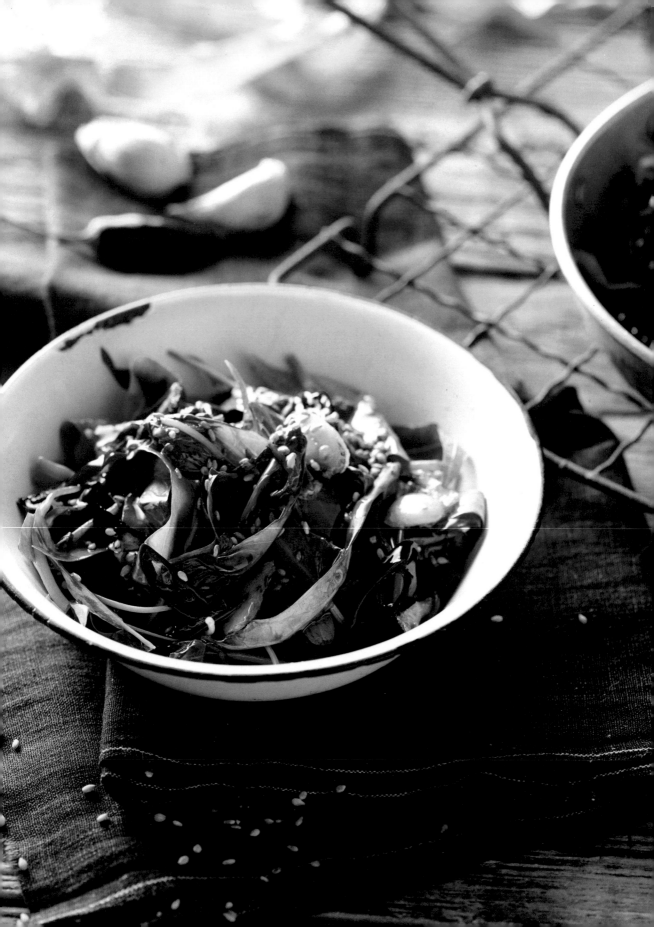

Water spinach, also know as *ong choy*, is a knockout when it comes to flavour and nutritional properties. It is high in magnesium, vitamins A and C, and is extremely high in fibre as well. Water spinach is a popular ingredient in Southeast Asia, where it is usually cooked with garlic and chillies and flavoured with fish sauce, vinegar, or soy sauce or any combination of these ingredients. It makes a great side dish to virtually any Asian-inspired dish that comes out of your wok, frying pan, oven, steamer, grill, or barbecue. If you cannot find water spinach, substitute regular spinach.

WATER SPINACH
WITH GARLIC & CHILLIES

SERVES 2 TO 4

2 tbsp coconut oil

2 fresh red chillies, chopped

2 cloves garlic, sliced

1 tsp shrimp paste

9 oz (250 g) water spinach or regular spinach, cut into 1¼-inch (3 cm) lengths

3 to 4 tbsp water or chicken stock (page 202)

White sesame seeds, toasted

Heat a wok over medium-high heat, add the coconut oil, and swirl it around until it melts and becomes hot. Add the chillies, garlic, and shrimp paste, and cook until it smells fragrant, 1 minute. Stir in the water spinach and water; toss and cook until the water spinach is just wilted, about 30 seconds. Season with sea salt and freshly cracked black pepper, and garnish with sesame seeds. Serve at once.

With the addition of sweet apples and carrots, this recipe is great for getting kids started on fermented foods – mine eat ½ teaspoon with their dinner each night, and they are even starting to enjoy it! You can even add a bit of the juice from the jar to a smoothie. When letting the sauerkraut ferment, the longer you leave it, the higher the level of good bacteria present. It's up to you how long; some people prefer the tangier flavour that comes from extra fermenting times, while others prefer a milder flavour. For more information on fermented foods, see page 9.

SAUERKRAUT
WITH CARROTS & APPLES
MAKES ABOUT 1½ QUARTS (1.5L)

14 oz (400 g) green cabbage

14 oz (400 g) red cabbage

2 red apples, cored

8 oz (250 g) carrots

1 packet (2 g to 5 g) vegetable culture starter (size varies depending on brand)

You will need a 1½-litre fermenting jar with airlock (I use a Culture For Life jar). Use very hot water to wash the jar as well as all utensils that will be used. Alternatively, you can run them through the hot rinse cycle in the dishwasher without adding any detergent.

Remove the outer leaves of the cabbage. Choose an unblemished one, wash it well, and then set aside for later.

Shred the cabbages, apples, and carrots in a food processor, alternating ingredients so they are all mixed together thoroughly. (You can also use a mandoline slicer or chop them by hand.) Transfer the vegetable mixture to a large glass or stainless steel mixing bowl.

Sprinkle 1½ tsp sea salt over the vegetables. Mix well and then cover with a plate while you activate the culture starter by mixing with filtered water according to the directions on the packet. Add the prepared culture starter to the bowl and mix again thoroughly.

Using a large spoon, fill the prepared fermenting jar with the mix, pressing down well between additions to remove any air pockets (a potato masher works well). Leave approximately ¾ inch (2 cm) of space free at the top. Your vegetables should be submerged in the liquid. If you don't have enough liquid, add more water until you do.

Take the reserved cabbage leaf, fold it, and place it on top of your vegetables. Add a small glass weight (a small shot glass is ideal) to keep everything submerged. Close with a lid fitted with an airlock to seal. Wrap a towel around the jar to block out any light, leaving the airlock exposed. (Note: If using a Culture For Life jar, the jar has a built-in system to keep the vegetables submerged. Simply place the jar into its silicone cover to block out the light.)

Place the jar in a dark, warm (60°F to 74°F/16°C to 23°C) spot – or in a portable cooler to maintain a more consistent temperature – and allow to culture for up to 2 weeks. The warmer the weather, the shorter the time it needs to ferment. After 1 week, taste it; the sauerkraut becomes more sour the longer you leave it, so when you are happy with the flavour and intensity, put the jar in the refrigerator to chill before eating. Once opened, it will last for up to 2 months in the fridge when kept submerged in the liquid. If unopened, it will keep for up to 9 months in the fridge.

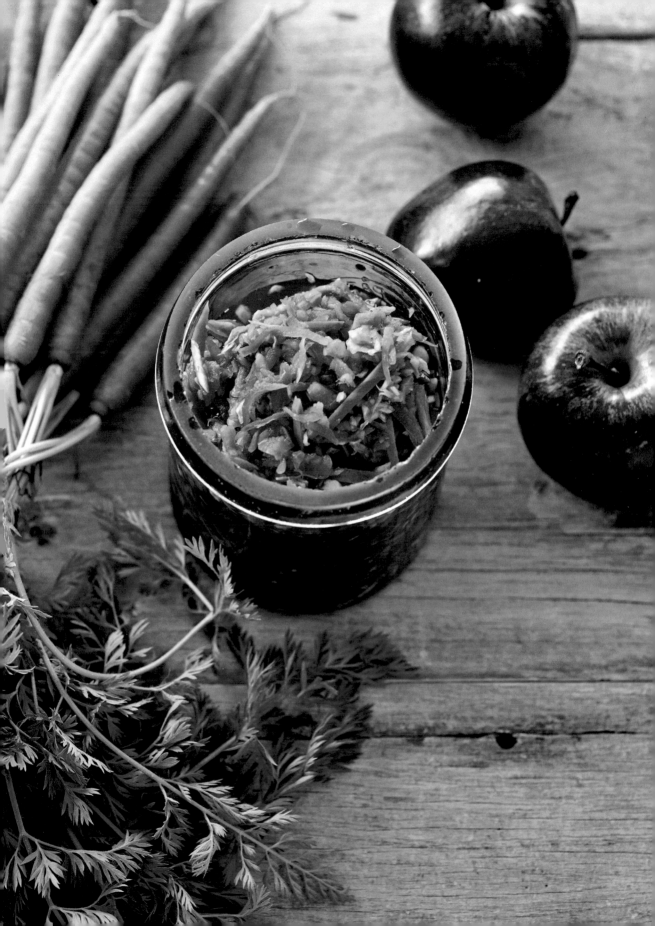

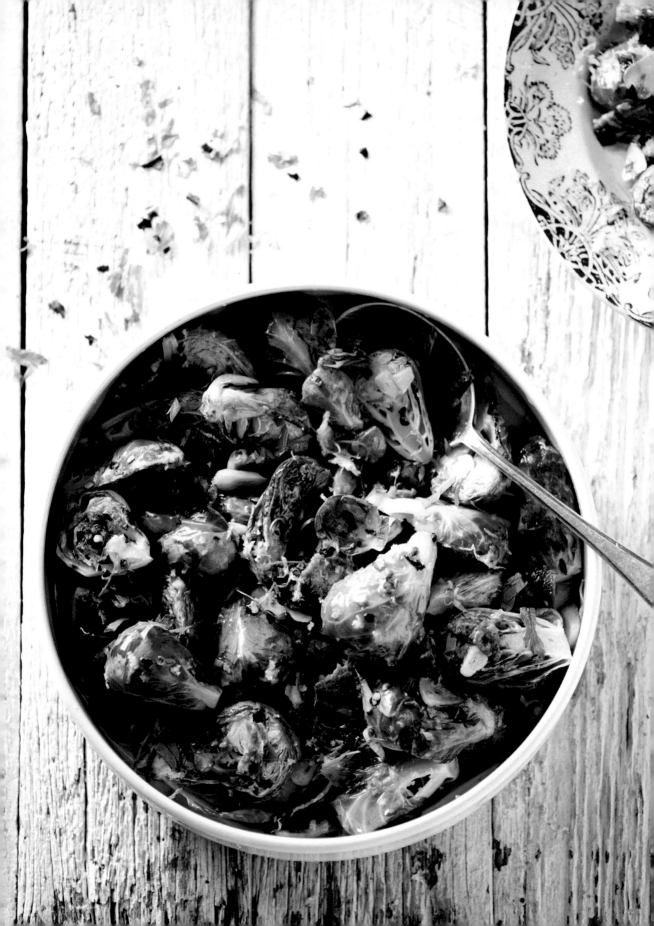

A member of the cruciferous vegetable family along with kale, cauliflower, and broccoli, Brussels sprouts are full of vitamins K, C, and A as well as loads of essential minerals. This recipe can be a game changer when it comes to kids or even adults enjoying them, especially for anyone who has horrid memories of having to eat overcooked soggy ones as a child. Here, they are combined with bacon and pan-fried with duck fat, which takes them to new culinary heights. They are perfect when served alongside pork, chicken, or even a steak.

BRUSSELS SPROUTS
WITH BACON & GARLIC
SERVES 4

⅓ cup (80 ml) duck fat, coconut oil, ghee, or lard

7 oz (200 g) good-quality bacon, coarsely chopped

1⅓ lb (600 g) Brussels sprouts, halved

6 cloves garlic, sliced

½ cup (60 ml) chicken stock (page 202)

Finely grated zest of 1 lemon

Red chilli flakes, to serve (optional)

Heat the duck fat in a large, heavy frying pan over medium heat. Add the bacon and cook, stirring occasionally, until the bacon starts to colour, 4 to 6 minutes. Add the Brussels sprouts and garlic for cook for 2 minutes or until the Brussels sprouts and garlic start to colour. Pour in the chicken stock and cook, stirring occasionally until the Brussels sprouts are tender, about 15 minutes.

To serve, sprinkle with lemon zest and red chilli flakes, if using.

I just love this dish – it is so perfect on a hot summer evening when you want something light to tuck into. Courgettes are primarily water and contain essential vitamins and minerals, but most of those are found in the skin, so never peel your courgettes. Because you don't peel them, be sure to source organic and locally grown whenever possible. The cheese layer in this dish is made from cashew or macadamia nut cheese, which makes it very scrumptious. Add some slices of smoked salmon or even liver pâté to the dish if you want a bit of added protein.

RAW COURGETTE LASAGNA
WITH TOMATO-OLIVE PESTO
SERVES 6

tomato-olive pesto
½ head broccoli florets (about 7 oz/200 g)

½ cup (60 g) pitted green Sicilian olives

3 vine-ripened tomatoes, seeded and chopped

7 oz (200 g) oil-packed sun-dried tomatoes, drained

7 oz (200 g) button mushrooms

2 cloves garlic, finely chopped

1 fresh red chilli, seeded and chopped

1 sprig rosemary, chopped

6 tbsp extra virgin olive oil

1 tbsp red wine vinegar

1 tbsp tomato paste

5 large courgettes

⅓ cup (80 ml) good-quality extra virgin olive oil, plus extra for brushing

1 bunch of basil leaves, torn

1 cup (220 g) cashew cheese (page 208)

2 tbsp freshly squeezed lemon juice

1 clove garlic, finely chopped

1 tbsp finely chopped fresh flat-leaf parsley

12 cherry tomatoes, quartered

Fresh baby purple and red basil leaves, to garnish (optional)

To make the pesto, combine the broccoli, olives, fresh and sun-dried tomatoes, mushrooms, garlic, chilli, rosemary, olive oil, vinegar and tomato paste in a food processor and process until smooth. Add a little water or oil, if needed, to make a spreadable paste. Season with sea salt and freshly cracked black pepper. Set aside.

To make the lasagna, slice the courgettes lengthwise on a mandoline or with a sharp knife to make sheets as thin as possible. Using a 5 by 9-inch (14 by 22 cm) loaf pan, lay 6 to 8 slices of courgette 'noodles' lengthwise in the pan, slightly overlapping to cover the dish. Brush with a little olive oil and sprinkle with a touch of salt. Evenly spread 8 tbsp of the pesto on the courgette layer, and then sprinkle with some torn basil. Add another layer of courgette slices and brush with a little olive oil and season with salt. Spread about 6 tbsp of the cashew cheese on the second layer of courgette, then evenly place another layer of courgette on top. Spread with another 6 tbsp of pesto and torn basil over the top. Repeat this process again, or until you have used up all the ingredients, but reserve some courgette for the top. Finally, lay the final layer of courgette, brush with a little oil, and season with salt.

Cover with plastic wrap and place in the freezer. Freeze for 2 hours or until frozen. This allows the lasagna to be cut into nice, neat portions. When the lasagna has frozen, remove it from the pan, cut it into six portions, and place in the fridge to thaw for 1 hour.

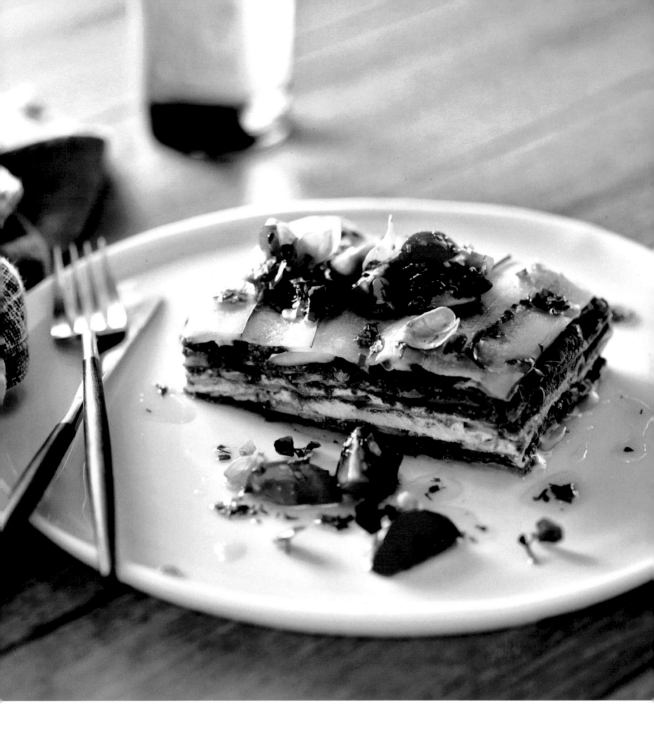

Just before serving, combine the lemon juice, remaining ⅓ cup (80 ml) olive oil, garlic, and parsley in a bowl and give it a good whisk to combine. Add the cherry tomatoes and toss. Season the tomatoes with salt and pepper.

Place the lasagna onto serving plates, top with the tomato salad, then drizzle any extra dressing from the tomato salad over the lasagna. Finish with some baby basil leaves, a pinch of salt, and some freshly cracked pepper.

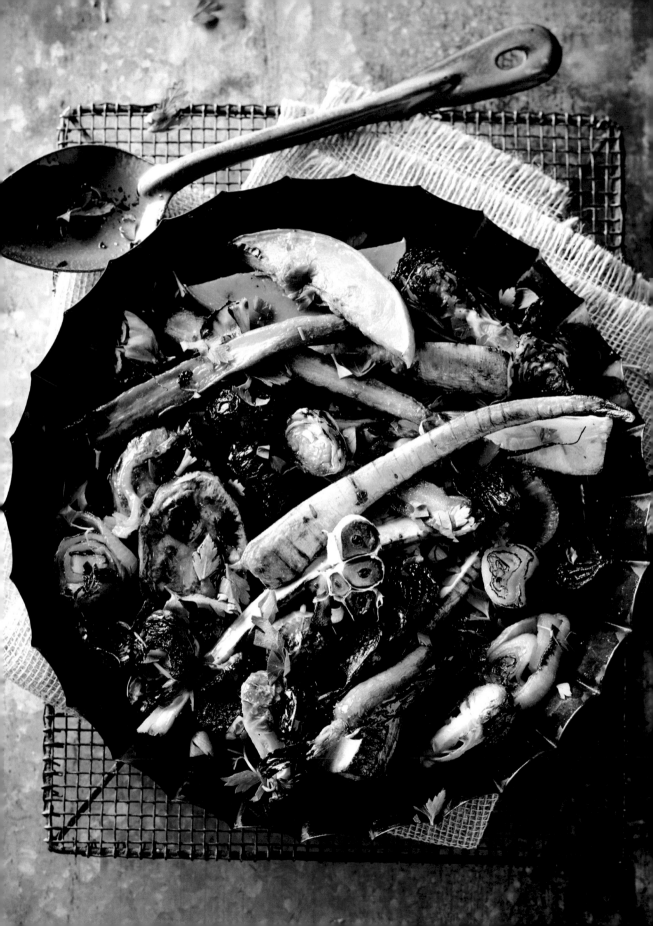

Slow-roasted vegetables are a favourite in my household, and I love to draw inspiration from around the globe to make different combinations by varying the veggies, herbs, and spices. Whether Brussels sprouts with lightly toasted nuts and bacon to serve with pork; simple slow-roasted tomatoes, olives, and thyme to serve with seafood; or one of my favourites – Jerusalem artichokes, kale, toasted almonds, and harissa to serve with a variety of meats . . . yum! The scrumptious recipe that follows uses 'a bit of everything', which is perfect for using up vegetables that are at the end of their tether in the fridge (I don't like wasting food).

ROASTED WINTER VEGETABLES
SERVES 4 TO 6

7 oz (200 g) parsnips (about 2), peeled and halved lengthwise

1 brown onion, quartered

¼ butternut squash, cut into small wedges

7 oz (200 g) sweet potato, peeled and sliced ½ inch (2 cm) thick

7 oz (200 g) Brussels sprouts, halved

7 oz (200 g) baby carrots (about ½ bunch), trimmed and peeled

5 oz (150 g) baby beetroots (about ½ bunch), trimmed, peeled, and halved

1 head garlic, halved crosswise across the cloves

4 tbsp melted duck fat, beef tallow, coconut oil, or ghee

4 tbsp coarsely chopped fresh flat-leaf parsley

Preheat the oven to 400°F (200°C gas 6). Combine the parsnips, onion, butternut squash, sweet potato, Brussels sprouts, baby carrots, baby beetroots, and garlic bulb in a large roasting tin and toss with the duck fat. Season with sea salt and freshly cracked black pepper. Spread out the vegetables into a single layer, making sure they're not bunched up together.

Roast until the vegetables are tender and golden, stirring once during cooking, 20 to 30 minutes. Squeeze the garlic out of its skin if you like and toss with the vegetables. Garnish with parsley and serve.

SEAFOOD

77
sardines escabeche

78
oysters with ginger
& spring onions

81
tuna tartare on nori crisps

82
smoked trout, kale
& fennel salad with
lime-chervil dressing

85
spicy tuna hand rolls

86
prawn laksa

89
poached prawns with
avocado-preserved
lemon salad

90
grilled wild salmon with
artichoke salsa

93
chorizo & seafood paella

94
grilled mackerel with smoky
chouriço salad

97
mussels with tomatoes,
leek & spicy saffron sauce

98
wild salmon with
beetroot salad & fennel

101
snapper en papillote with
clams & cherry tomatoes

102
wild salmon with coconut-lime
sauce & sweet potato puree

105
seafood curry

106
fish & chips

109
prawn satay

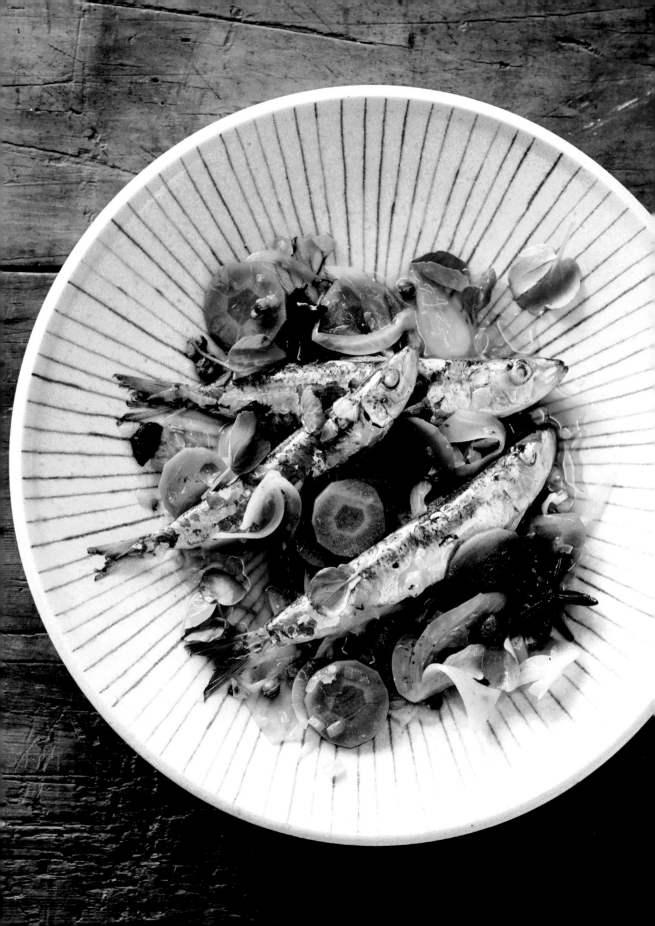

The sheer deliciousness of sardines, their incredible health benefits, and the fact that they're so darn easy to prepare definitely earns them a prize in my book. Consider their nutritional benefits: one 3-ounce (75 g) serving of sardines supplies more than 120 percent of the recommended daily intake of vitamin B_{12}, roughly 60 percent of the required daily selenium intake, 50 percent of the daily protein, 40 percent of daily vitamin D, and 35 percent of daily calcium needs. My number-one sardine preparation is *escabeche*, which originated in Spain and Portugal. Use a premium vinegar to cut through the richness of the lively sardine. To really make this dish special, prepare it a few days in advance to allow the sardines to bathe in the flavours.

SARDINES ESCABECHE
SERVES 4

1 tsp coriander seeds, lightly crushed

½ tsp cumin seeds, lightly crushed

12 sardines, fins and bones removed (if you like them boneless; I don't mind the bones to munch on), heads and tails intact

3 tbsp coconut oil

1 red onion, thinly sliced

1 fennel bulb, shaved

1 carrot, peeled and thinly sliced

1 clove garlic, finely chopped

1 cup (250 ml) white wine or verjus

1½ cups (375 ml) raw apple cider vinegar

2 bay leaves

2 sprigs thyme

2 star anise

Pinch of saffron

2 tbsp baby capers

2 large handfuls of watercress

Toast the coriander and cumin seeds in a frying pan over medium heat until golden and fragrant, about 30 seconds. Remove the spices from the pan, transfer to a mortar, and coarsely grind with a pestle.

Rinse the sardines and pat dry. Wipe the pan clean with a paper towel and return the pan to the stove over medium heat. Add 1 tbsp coconut oil and pan-fry the sardines for 1 minute on each side; do this in batches if necessary. Transfer to a wide, heatproof container in a single layer. Add the remaining 2 tbsp oil to the pan and cook the onion, fennel, carrot, garlic, and ground toasted spices until the vegetables are transparent but not browned, 3 to 5 minutes. Lightly season with sea salt and freshly cracked black pepper. Add the wine, vinegar, bay leaves, thyme, star anise, and saffron to the pan. Bring to a boil, reduce the heat, and simmer for 5 minutes. Remove from the heat and let stand for 10 minutes to cool slightly.

Ladle the warm pickling liquid and vegetables over the sardines, making sure the sardines are completely submerged in the liquid. Allow to cool completely. Cover and transfer to the refrigerator to marinate for at least 12 hours and up to 48 hours for the flavour to develop.

To serve, remove the bay leaves, thyme sprigs, and star anise and arrange the sardines on a large platter or four serving plates. Spoon the pickling liquid and vegetables over the sardines and garnish with capers and watercress.

I love oysters so much, I am writing an entire book dedicated to this marvel of the ocean with a good mate of mine – a professional oyster shucker for the last thirty years. This recipe is a classic Chinese preparation. The key here is to first slice the ginger paper thin, and then cut it into fine long strands; the same goes for the spring onions. The sauce is a combination of vinegar and tamari; you can use coconut aminos or fish sauce instead of tamari if you prefer. When I substitute fish sauce, I like to add a touch of finely chopped fresh red chilli, lime juice, and some chopped lemongrass.

OYSTERS
WITH GINGER & SPRING ONIONS
SERVES 2

sauce

1-inch (3 cm) piece fresh ginger, peeled and julienned

⅓ cup (80 ml) wheat-free tamari or coconut aminos

¼ cup (60 ml) fish stock (page 202) or water

1 tbsp raw apple cider vinegar

12 oysters, in the half shell, ideally local

4 spring onions, julienned

to serve

Toasted sesame oil

Fresh coriander leaves

Fresh shiso leaves

White sesame seeds, toasted

To make the sauce, combine the ginger, tamari, fish stock, and vinegar in a small saucepan over a medium heat. Heat to a simmer for 2 minutes, then remove from the heat and set aside.

Place the oysters in a steaming basket set over boiling water and spoon a good amount of sauce on each. Add a small amount of spring onions to each one. Cover the pan with its lid and steam for 1 to 2 minutes. Drizzle with some of the remaining sauce after steaming.

To finish, drizzle the oysters with sesame oil and garnish with coriander, shiso, and sesame seeds.

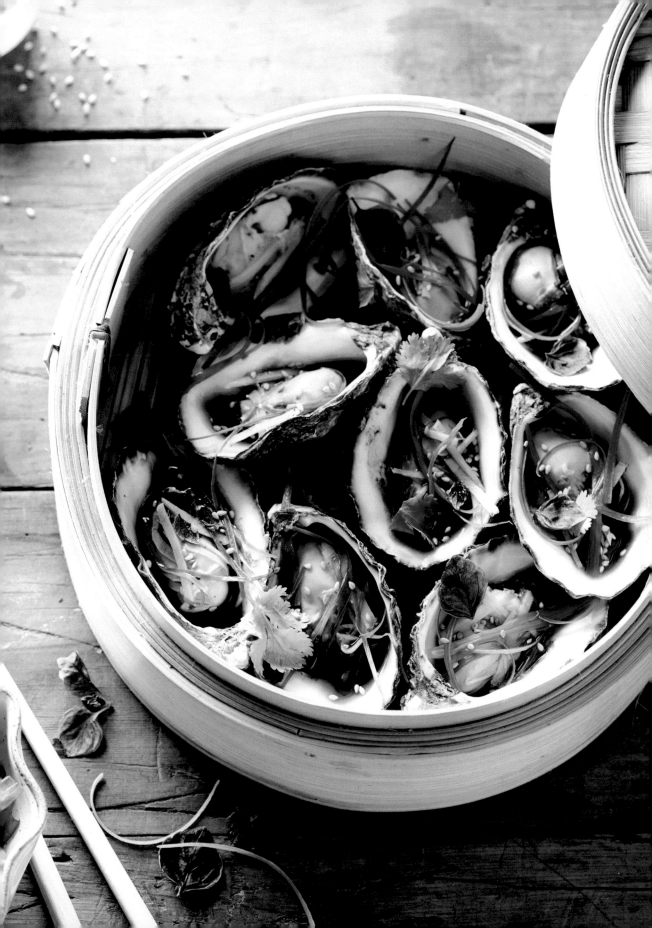

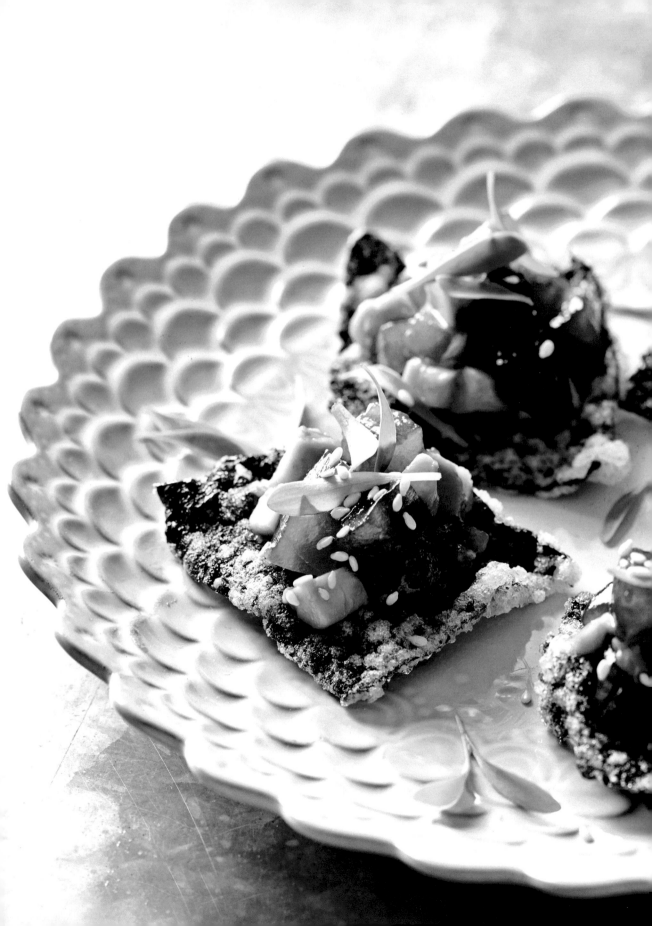

These yummy little bite-size canapés were a hit over the holidays. I served them before we sat down for our Christmas lunch, and everyone absolutely loved them. The inspiration for this dish came from an incredible chef named Ravi Kapur. Ravi and I worked together on Outstanding in the Field, a pop-up restaurant series that was founded in Santa Cruz, California, and he made a version of these that rocked my world so much I just had to construct my own rendition. This recipe is beautiful with different types of fresh fish and seafood, especially salmon, prawns, scallops, or one of my ultimate favourites: sea urchin.

TUNA TARTARE ON NORI CRISPS

MAKES 18 BITES

nori crisps
1½ cups (150 g) tapioca flour

⅔ cup (150 ml) ice-cold soda water

Melted coconut oil, for frying

3 nori sheets, each cut into 6 even squares

tuna tartare
9 oz (250 g) best-quality sashimi-grade tuna

½ avocado, peeled and pitted

1 tbsp toasted sesame oil

1 tbsp peeled and grated fresh ginger

2 tbsp yuzu juice

2 tbsp wheat-free tamari or coconut aminos

½ tsp chilli oil (optional)

2 tbsp lemon-infused olive oil

1 tsp toasted white sesame seeds

Fresh baby coriander leaves, to garnish

To make the nori crisps, put the tapioca flour in a mixing bowl and slowly pour in the soda water while you whisk. Continue whisking until the batter has the consistency of single cream.

Add oil to a depth of 4 inches (10 cm) to a wok or deep saucepan. Heat the oil to 320°F (160°C). Dip each nori sheet, one at a time, into the batter to coat completely, then slide it straight into the hot oil. (The nori sheet will become very soft very quickly once it is covered in the batter, so it's best to put it straight into the frying oil after coating. Do this in batches.) Fry the nori on both sides until light and golden, about 30 seconds. Drain on paper towels and sprinkle with sea salt.

To make the tartare, dice the tuna into small pieces and place in a chilled bowl. Dice the avocado into the same size as the tuna and add to the tuna with sesame oil, ginger, yuzu juice, tamari, chilli oil, if using, and lemon oil. Mix until combined and season with salt and freshly cracked black pepper.

Spoon a tsp of the tuna mix on a nori crisp, and sprinkle with some toasted sesame seeds and coriander. Repeat until all the crisps and tartare are used.

Fishing for wild trout is one of my favourite things to do, alone or with the family. To be able to go into the wilderness and walk upstream and cast for your next meal is very special. And it doesn't get any fresher than that! In addition, you know that the fish has had a natural diet of smaller fish, insects, or crustaceans that also live in the river. Freshwater fish are milder in flavour than their ocean-dwelling cousins, so an added pinch of quality salt or other spice or seasoning is often needed. Here is a great salad that you can add pretty much any seafood to, although I do love the texture and flavour of good-quality smoked trout.

SMOKED TROUT, KALE & FENNEL SALAD
WITH LIME-CHERVIL DRESSING

SERVES 4

dressing
¼ cup (60 ml) extra virgin olive oil

2½ tbsp freshly squeezed lime juice

1 tbsp raw apple cider vinegar

1 tbsp chopped fresh chervil

1 fresh red chilli, seeded and finely chopped

salad
½ bunch of kale, tough stems removed and leaves shredded

3 tbsp extra virgin olive oil

¼ head red cabbage, shredded

1 fennel bulb, shaved

1 red onion, thinly sliced

1 large handful of lamb's lettuce

1 hot-smoked rainbow trout, skin and bones removed and flesh flaked

¾ cup (120 g) almonds, activated (page 209) and chopped

To make the dressing, whisk together the olive oil, lime juice, vinegar, chervil, and chilli in a bowl. Season with sea salt and freshly cracked black pepper and set aside.

To make the salad, put the kale in a large bowl and pour the olive oil over it. Rub the oil into the kale with your hands, almost like you are massaging the kale. This removes the waxy coating from the kale and allows it to absorb the dressing. Pour the dressing over the kale, toss, and leave to stand for at least 30 minutes before serving.

Just before serving, add the cabbage, fennel, onion, lamb's lettuce, and trout and gently toss. Transfer to a large platter and sprinkle with the almonds.

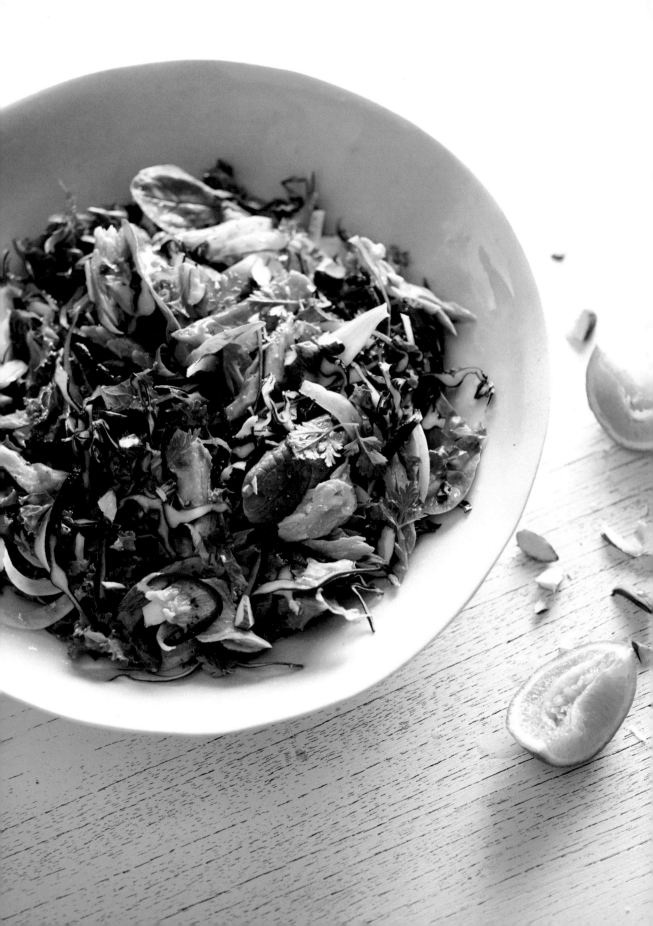

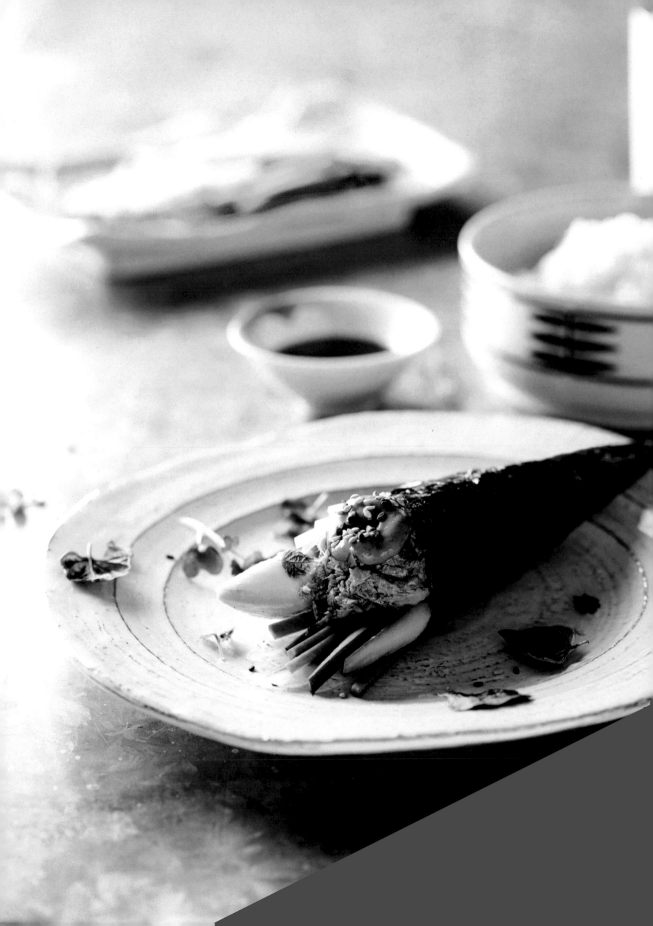

Since becoming a father, I've learned to never underestimate how much kids love to help out in the kitchen, even if just to set the table (folding napkins is fun!), because it gives them a sense of achievement that they are contributing to the family meal. This is one of our family's favourite recipes. We all sit around the table with bowls of assorted ingredients in the centre – fresh raw fish, seaweed, kimchi, raw vegetables, toasted sesame seeds, avocado, Cauliflower Rice (page 61), and wasabi – and make the rolls together. I love watching the kids create their own wonderful combinations.

SPICY TUNA HAND ROLLS
SERVES 4 TO 6

6 tbsp mayonnaise (page 203)

3 tsp fermented hot chilli sauce (page 205)

1 tsp peeled and grated fresh ginger

⅛ tsp hot sesame oil, or to taste

1 (12 oz/340 g) can tuna packed in water, drained

About 1 cup (200 g) Cauliflower Rice (page 61)

6 toasted nori sheets

1 avocado, peeled, pitted, and sliced

½ cucumber, cut into matchsticks

½ carrot, cut into matchsticks

2½-inch (6.25 cm) piece mooli, thinly julienned

Small handful of baby shiso leaves

1 tbsp each black and white sesame seeds, toasted

Wheat-free tamari or coconut aminos, to serve

Wasabi, to serve

To make the spicy tuna, stir together the mayonnaise, hot chilli sauce, ginger, and hot sesame oil in a serving bowl. Add the tuna and cauliflower rice and mix together well. Refrigerate for 5 minutes to set.

Cut the nori sheets in halves, forming 4 by 7-inch (10 by 18 cm) pieces. Place a nori piece in the palm of your hand, shiny side down, and top with some of the spicy tuna mixture, avocado, cucumber, carrot, mooli, and shiso leaves. Fold a bottom corner of the nori over the filling and then roll up to form a cone shape. Sprinkle over some sesame seeds. Repeat to make 12 rolls. Serve immediately with the tamari as a dipping sauce and the wasabi.

Laksa is a dish that keeps you coming back for more. One of the main ingredients is turmeric, which is a super food. Even though it's a humble and unassuming ingredient, it is a spice that has been used for centuries. Ancient doctors and modern-day scientists alike agree that this little yellow rhizome, which has both anti-fungal and anti-inflammatory characteristics, packs a nutritional punch. I like to use both fresh and powdered turmeric. The most obvious use for turmeric is as the base for an aromatic curry paste. I have used kelp noodles in this dish instead of the standard rice or egg noodles; however, you can omit them completely and just use more vegetables if you like.

PRAWN LAKSA
SERVES 4

9 oz (250 g) kelp noodles

6 cloves garlic

7 oz (200 g) fresh red chillies, coarsely chopped

2 lemongrass stalks, white part only, thinly sliced

5 kaffir lime leaves, finely shredded

1 tsp ground turmeric

3 (15¼ oz/440 ml) cans coconut milk

2 tbsp raw honey

1 tsp tamarind concentrate

1 lb (500 g) king prawns, peeled, tails intact, and de-veined

3 tbsp fish sauce

3 tbsp freshly squeezed lime juice

¼ head Chinese cabbage, finely shredded

to serve

1 handful of bean sprouts

½ bunch of Thai basil, leaves only

1 small handful of fresh coriander leaves

Fried shallots (page 207)

Chilli oil

2 limes, halved

Soak the noodles in a bowl of cold water for 10 minutes to slightly soften, then drain.

Meanwhile, combine the garlic, chillies, lemongrass, lime leaves, and turmeric in a food processor and process into a paste, or pound using a mortar and pestle.

Bring the coconut milk to a boil over medium heat in a large, heavy saucepan. When it starts to boil, add the blended spice paste, honey, and tamarind and stir well. Add the prawns, return to a boil, then turn off the heat and let it sit until the prawns are just cooked through, 5 minutes. Add the fish sauce, lime juice, and cabbage. Turn the heat back on to medium and cook for 1 minute, then remove from the heat.

To serve, divide the noodles and prawns among four bowls. Spoon the sauce over and garnish with the bean sprouts, basil leaves, coriander, and fried shallots. Drizzle with the chilli oil. Serve with lime halves.

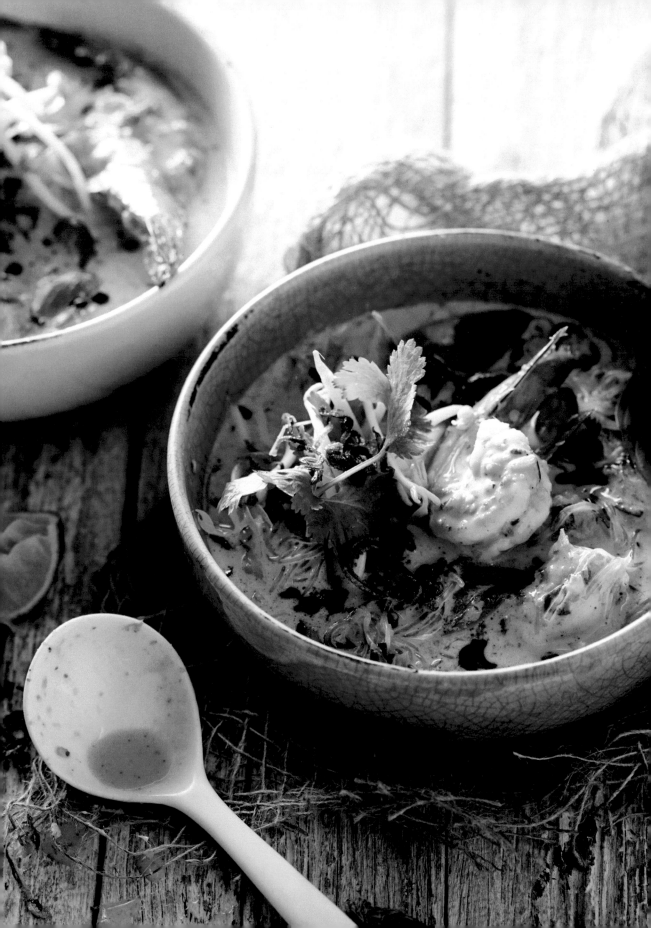

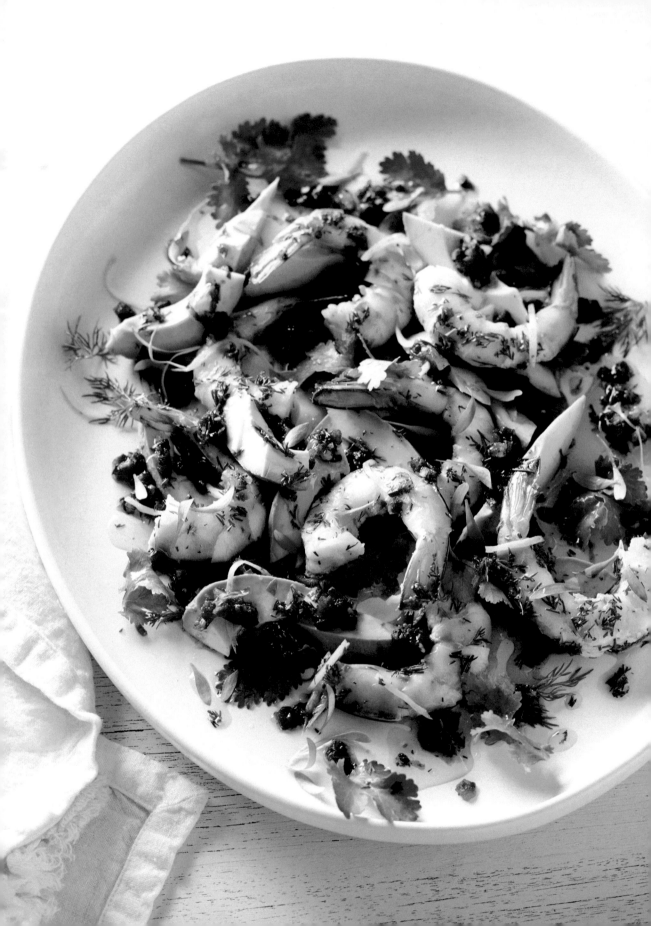

Prawns and avocado. I don't think there is a better combination of ingredients; in fact, it almost feels like you are cheating whenever you combine them because the results are so spectacular. Always source the freshest, plumpest prawns you can get your hands on. Find some gorgeous ripe avocados, juicy tomato, and fresh coriander and then transform these ingredients into a fresh salad that has a unique twist: preserved lemon. Sometimes I like to throw Sauerkraut (page 66) in as well. It will have your guests or family thinking you have spent hours in the kitchen.

POACHED PRAWNS
WITH AVOCADO–PRESERVED LEMON SALAD
SERVES 4

16 raw king prawns

3 tbsp lemon-infused extra virgin olive oil

1 tbsp freshly squeezed lemon juice

1 tsp chopped fresh dill

avocado salad

2 avocados, peeled, pitted and sliced

½ roasted red pepper (page 208), seeded and finely chopped

1 plum tomato, seeded and finely diced

1 bird's eye chilli, seeded and finely chopped

¼ red onion, finely diced

1 tbsp finely chopped preserved lemon rind

1 tbsp chopped fresh coriander

2 tbsp freshly squeezed lemon juice

2 tbsp lemon-infused extra virgin olive oil, plus more for drizzling

2 tbsp minced red pepper, for serving

1 handful of fresh coriander and dill leaves, for serving

Cook the prawns in salted boiling water until pink and firm, 2 to 3 minutes. Transfer to a bowl of ice-cold water and leave until the prawns are completely cold. Peel and de-vein, keeping the tails intact.

In a mixing bowl, combine the lemon olive oil, lemon juice, and dill and season with sea salt and freshly cracked black pepper. Whisk to combine, then add the prawns and toss until well coated. Marinate for 5 minutes in the refrigerator.

Meanwhile, make the avocado salad. Gently mix together the avocado, roasted red pepper, tomato, chilli, onion, preserved lemon, coriander, lemon juice, 2 tbsp of the lemon olive oil, and salt and pepper in a bowl.

Spoon the salad onto a serving platter and top with the marinated prawns. Garnish with the diced red pepper, fresh coriander and dill, and a drizzle of lemon olive oil, and serve.

I eat only wild salmon, and never farmed salmon. Followers of Paleo and lovers of the ocean do not condone farmed salmon because it isn't a natural way for the fish to live; not only that, but the amount of omega-6 fatty acids in farmed fish is higher and their omega-3 levels are lower, making farmed fish a less healthy option. Wild salmon is more expensive because fishermen can't compete with the prices of farmed salmon, so it's more important than ever to stand up for the greater good and support mindful fishermen who fish sustainably. You can substitute just about any sustainable fish for the salmon in this recipe and it will still be awesome. This is a gorgeous recipe that can be whipped up in minutes, and the taste is sublime. The artichoke salsa is even great on grilled lamb chops.

GRILLED WILD SALMON
WITH ARTICHOKE SALSA
SERVES 4

5½ oz (150 g) vine-ripened tomatoes, seeded and quartered

1 (3½ oz/100 g) jar marinated artichokes, drained

⅔ cup (80 g) pitted kalamata olives

1 handful of fresh flat-leaf parsley, chopped

¼ cup (30 g) pine nuts, activated (page 209) and toasted

⅔ cup (150 ml) extra virgin olive oil

Juice of 1 lemon

4 (6 oz/170 g) wild salmon steaks

Melted coconut oil, ghee, or duck fat, for cooking

Fresh baby basil leaves, to garnish

To make the salsa, finely dice the tomatoes and artichokes and place in a bowl. Add the olives, parsley, and pine nuts. Then add the olive oil and lemon juice and season with sea salt and freshly cracked black pepper. Set aside.

Preheat a grill pan to high or prepare a hot fire in a barbecue.

Brush the salmon with coconut oil, season with salt and pepper, and cook for a few minutes on each side, depending on how thick the fish is. Serve, topped with the salsa and garnished with the basil.

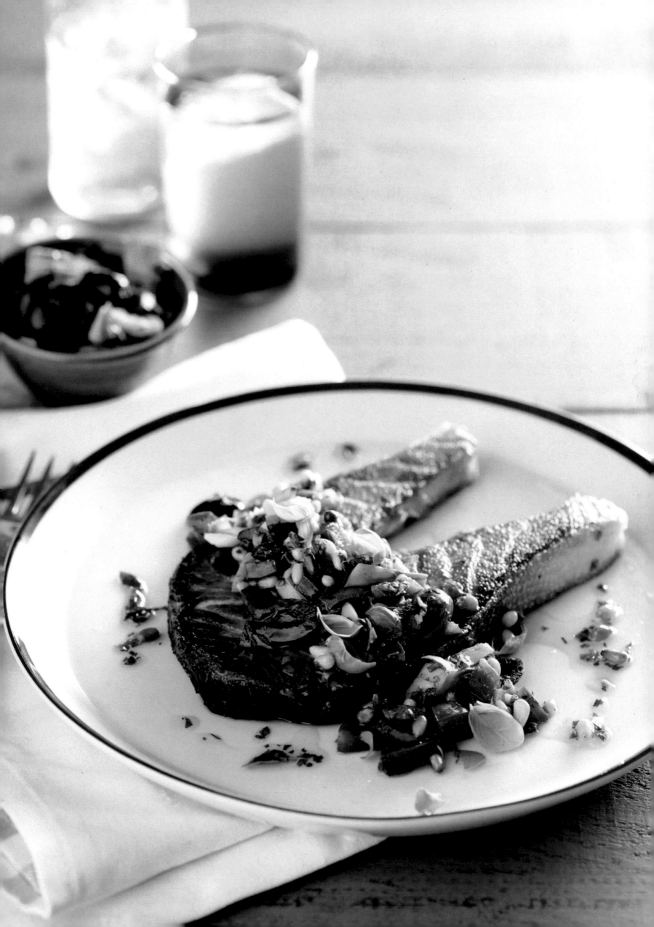

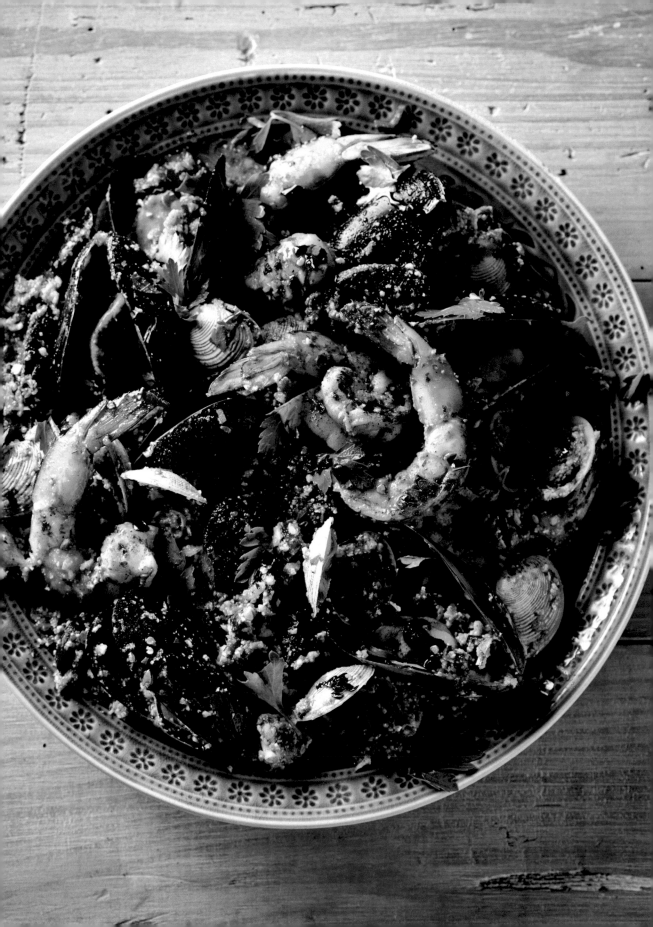

Spain is regarded as being at the forefront of the modern culinary movement, and a lot of chefs from around the world, including myself, make pilgrimages to this wonderful country to experience the most creative kitchens in the world. Some people may think it sacrilege to change rice, the main ingredient in paella, to cauliflower. However, one of the fathers of modernist cuisine, Ferran Adrià, from the former elBulli restaurant in Roses, Spain, reinvented couscous by cutting cauliflower into match head-sized pieces so that it resembled tiny couscous grains. This version of paella captures the essence of a great paella — without rice. I hope you enjoy this modern approach to a classic.

CHORIZO & SEAFOOD PAELLA
SERVES 4 TO 6

2 cups (500 ml) chicken stock (page 202)

2 pinches of saffron threads (15 to 20 threads)

1 head cauliflower, coarsely chopped

2 tbsp ghee or coconut oil

5 oz (150 g) Spanish chorizo, thickly sliced

2 red peppers, seeded and diced

2 fresh tomatoes, diced

1 large onion, chopped

4 cloves garlic, finely chopped

1 tbsp tomato paste

1 tsp sweet paprika

1 tbsp smoked paprika, plus more to serve

1 small bunch of fresh flat-leaf parsley, leaves and stems chopped separately

8 king prawns, peeled, with tails intact, and de-veined

14 oz (400 g) mussels, cleaned

10 oz (300 g) clams, cleaned

Extra virgin olive oil, for drizzling

½ lemon, juiced

Pour the stock into a saucepan, place over medium heat, and bring to a simmer. Remove from the heat, stir in the saffron threads, and set aside to infuse for 5 to 10 minutes.

Meanwhile, put the cauliflower in a food processor and process into tiny pieces resembling grains of rice. Set aside.

Heat the ghee in a large frying pan over medium heat, add the chorizo, and fry until golden and crispy, turning once, about 1 minute. Add the red peppers, tomatoes, onion, garlic, tomato paste, and sweet and smoked paprika and cook until the vegetables are soft, 2 to 3 minutes. Pour in the warm stock, add the parsley stems, and bring a boil. Add the prawns, mussels, and clams; place a lid on the pan and cook until the mussels and clams are open and the prawns are cooked, 2 to 3 minutes. Add the cauliflower, cook for 1 minute, and season with sea salt and freshly cracked black pepper.

To serve, transfer to a serving bowl. Garnish with the parsley leaves, drizzle with olive oil and lemon juice, and sprinkle with smoked paprika.

Doc Willoughby and Chris Schlesinger are respected American chefs with whom I had the good fortune to work for on a cooking series I was hosting. Doc and Chris took me clamming to start off our day checking out New England seafood. After raking the sand for a while, it was back to Chris's house to cook up a feast. My favourite dish of the day, however, was spanking-fresh blue mackerel that was partnered with a *chouriço* salad filled with ripe tomatoes, fresh herbs, a good glug of olive oil, and a splash of lemon juice, which helped cut through the rich chorizo and gave the fish the acid it loves. Thanks, fellas. It was a treat cooking and quahogging with you!

GRILLED MACKEREL
WITH SMOKY CHOURIÇO SALAD
SERVES 4

smoky chouriço salad
1 lb (450 g) *chouriço* (Portuguese chorizo) or Spanish chorizo, cut in half lengthwise

12 cherry tomatoes, quartered

⅓ cup (20 g) chopped fresh flat-leaf parsley

1 tbsp finely chopped garlic

¼ cup (60 ml) extra virgin olive oil

1 tbsp finely grated lemon zest

2 tbsp freshly squeezed lemon juice

1 tsp cumin seeds, lightly toasted

mackerel
4 (6⅓ oz/180 g) mackerel fillets, skin on

2 tbsp coconut oil, melted

Fresh baby basil leaves, to garnish

Prepare a barbecue or grill pan over medium-low heat.

To make the salad, grill the sausage until browned and warmed through, 3 to 4 minutes per side. Remove it from the barbecue or grill pan, dice it into small cubes, and put it into a bowl. Add the tomatoes, parsley, garlic, olive oil, lemon zest, lemon juice, and cumin seeds and toss to combine. Season the salad with sea salt and freshly cracked black pepper.

To prepare the mackerel, season the fillets with salt and pepper and rub them on both sides with the coconut oil. Put them skin side up on the barbecue or grill pan and cover them with foil. Cook until golden brown, about 5 minutes; remove the foil; and flip the fillets with a spatula. Cook the fish until completely opaque throughout and the skin is crisp, about 5 minutes more.

Remove the fillets from the barbecue or grill pan, place them on a platter, and serve them topped with the salad and garnished with baby basil.

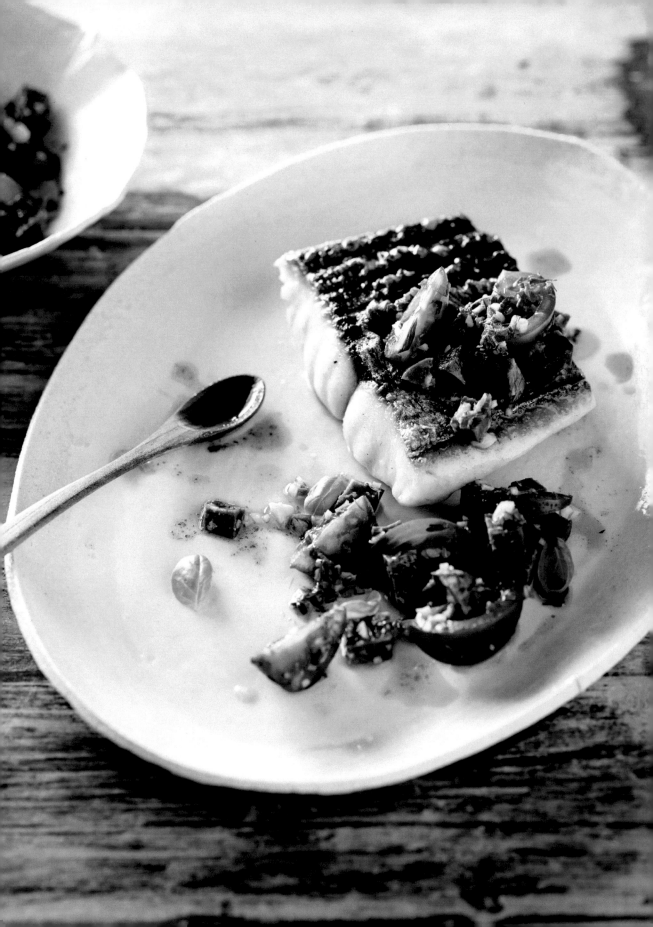

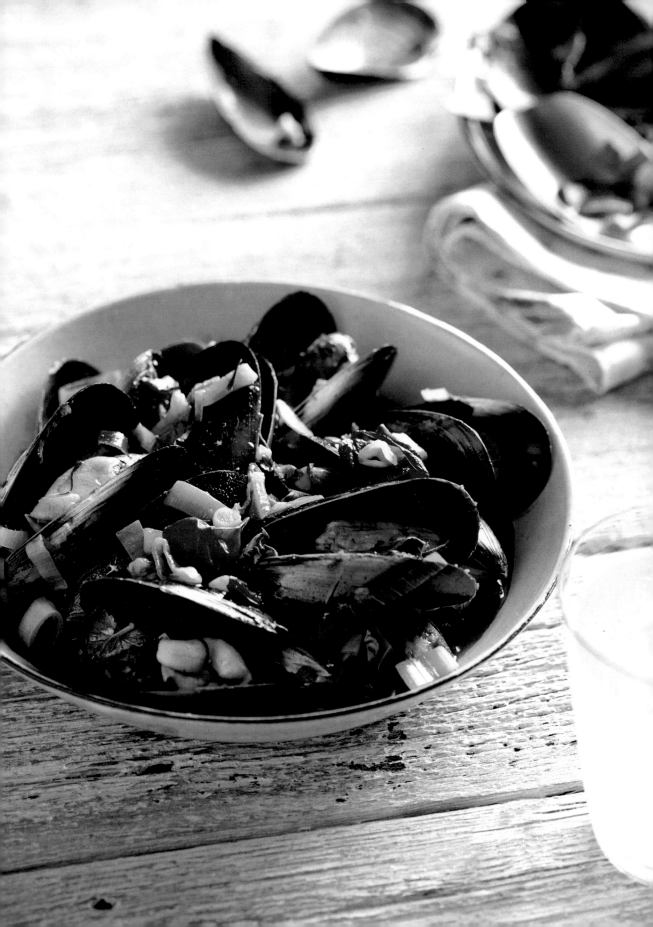

When you cook fresh mussels, you will find that they release a lot of their juices into the pan. You can strain some of this out (and then use it to flavour other seafood soups or stews) or keep it in, which will enhance your dish. Just be careful to take the mussels out as soon as they open to keep them from overcooking. Then you can continue reducing the broth or sauce to the desired consistency; after that, just toss the mussels back in to coat them. This is a wonderful, flavourful recipe that works great as a starter popped into a large bowl and served family-style in the middle of the table.

MUSSELS
WITH TOMATOES, LEEK & SPICY SAFFRON SAUCE
SERVES 2

4 tbsp ghee or coconut oil

3 cloves garlic, sliced

1 fresh red chilli, sliced

½ leek, white and tender green parts, halved lengthwise and sliced

1 tsp smoked paprika

¾ cup (175 ml) white wine

2 pinches of saffron threads (15 to 20 threads)

1 cup (250 ml) chicken stock (page 202)

2 spring onions, coarsely chopped

15 cherry tomatoes, halved

2 tbsp freshly squeezed lemon juice

2¼ lb (1 kg) mussels, scrubbed

1 large handful of fresh coriander leaves

Melt the ghee in a large pan over medium-high heat. Add the garlic, chilli, leek, and paprika and sauté until fragrant, 1 minute. Add the wine and saffron. Simmer for 5 minutes, then add the chicken stock, spring onions, tomatoes, and lemon juice. Simmer until the tomatoes are soft and starting to blister, 5 minutes.

Add the mussels, cover the pan, and cook until they are open, 4 to 5 minutes. Shake the pan, holding down the lid with a tea towel, to redistribute the mussels. Discard any mussels that do not open. Add the handful of coriander and mix in with the mussels.

To serve, divide the mussels between two bowls. Pour over the broth, distributing it equally among the bowls, and serve.

I have cooked for some well-known people, from royalty to celebrities. But I was more nervous about cooking for Nora Gedgaudas than any of the others! Nora, author of the must-read *Primal Body, Primal Mind*, is one of the most influential leaders in the Paleo/primal movement. This is the dish I cooked for her because it includes healthy omega-3s from wild salmon, a powerhouse of nutrients from beetroots and pomegranates, and calcium from the tahini.

WILD SALMON
WITH BEETROOT SALAD & FENNEL
SERVES 4

beetroot salad
Coconut oil, melted, for greasing

12 oz (320 g) beetroots, peeled and diced into ¼-inch (5 mm) cubes

½ cup (80 g) black quinoa, rinsed (optional)

2 tbsp red wine vinegar

¼ tsp ground cumin

½ tsp ground sumac

1 clove garlic, finely chopped

4 tbsp extra virgin olive oil

Seeds of 1 pomegranate

3 tbsp each chopped fresh mint and coriander leaves

tahini sauce
2 tbsp unhulled tahini paste

1 tbsp extra virgin olive oil

1 clove garlic, finely chopped

Juice of 1 lemon

quick braised fennel
1 tbsp ghee or coconut oil

2 fennel bulbs, shaved

⅓ cup (80 ml) lemon-infused extra virgin olive oil

Juice of 1 lemon

fish
4 (6 oz/170 g) wild salmon fillets, skin on, pin bones removed

2 tbsp coconut oil, melted

to serve
3 tbsp pistachio nuts, activated (page 209), roasted, and coarsely chopped

Fennel fronds, roughly torn

Pomegranate molasses

Preheat the oven to 400°F (200°C gas 6). Grease a baking sheet with coconut oil, then add the beetroots in a single layer. Season with sea salt and freshly cracked black pepper and cover with aluminium foil. Bake for 15 minutes. Remove from the oven and let cool. If making quinoa, add it to a saucepan with 2½ cups (600 ml) water. Place over medium-high heat, bring to a boil, and cook until tender, 10 minutes. Drain and cool. In a bowl, whisk together the vinegar, cumin, sumac, garlic, and olive oil. Combine the beetroots, quinoa, pomegranate seeds, mint, and coriander in a bowl. Drizzle with the dressing, season with salt and pepper, and toss well.

To make the tahini sauce, in a small bowl, whisk together the tahini paste, olive oil, garlic, lemon juice, and 1 tbsp water. Set aside. To make the braised fennel, heat a frying pan with the ghee over medium-low heat. Add the fennel and ¼ cup (60 ml) water and cook, stirring, until the fennel is just tender, 3 minutes. Strain out any liquid. Let the fennel cool then add the lemon olive oil and lemon juice. Season with salt and pepper and set aside.

To prepare the fish, coat the salmon with 1 tbsp coconut oil and season with salt and pepper. Heat the remaining 1 tbsp oil in a frying pan over medium-high heat. Add the fish, skin side down, and cook until the skin is golden, 2 to 3 minutes. Turn and cook until the fish is medium-rare, 2 minutes. Transfer the fish to a plate, tent with foil, and let rest for 2 minutes. To serve, divide the tahini sauce among four plates. Top each with fennel, then place the fish on top. Add the beetroot salad and sprinkle with pistachio nuts, then finish with fennel fronds and a drizzle of pomegranate molasses.

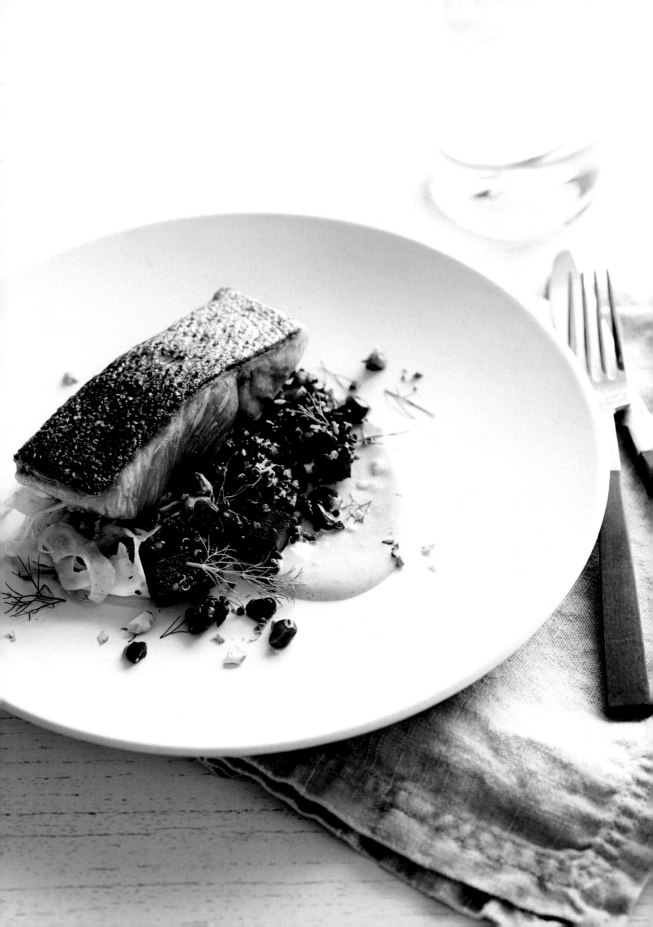

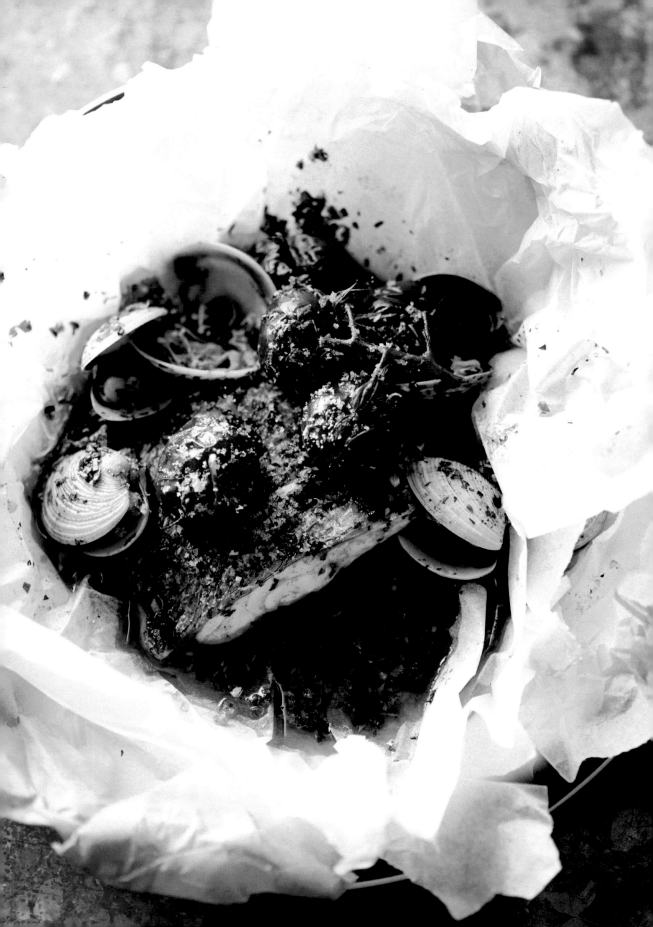

It's no secret that I absolutely love cooking, but I don't always have a lot of time, so occasionally I have to get in and out of the kitchen quickly. If you're in the same boat from time to time, then this is the recipe for you! It's so quick and easy to prepare – and nutritious and delicious as well. This recipe has a Mediterranean feel to it, with ripe fresh tomatoes to add acidity and sweetness and tender clams to top it off beautifully. Serve this with a gorgeous plate of green veggies or a simple salad.

SNAPPER EN PAPILLOTE
WITH CLAMS & CHERRY TOMATOES
SERVES 2

2 (6⅓ oz/180 g) snapper or sea bass fillets

10 clams, cleaned

2 tbsp finely chopped garlic

¾ cup (100 g) ghee or coconut oil, melted

4 tbsp chopped fresh flat-leaf parsley

1 tbsp diced fresh red chilli

⅓ cup (80 ml) dry white wine

10 cherry tomatoes

Zest and juice of 1 lemon

1 tsp grated bottarga (see Note below)

Preheat the oven to 425°F (220°C gas 7). In a large deep roasting pan, place two large sheets of baking parchment side by side; each piece should be large enough to enclose half the fish and clams.

Season the fish with sea salt and freshly cracked black pepper and place one fillet in the centre of each piece of parchment. In a bowl, mix together the clams, garlic, ghee, parsley, chilli, wine, tomatoes, lemon zest and juice, and spoon over the fish, dividing the ingredients evenly. Fold each piece of baking parchment over from both sides to form a package, tucking in the ends to seal. Bake until the fish is cooked through and the clams open, about 10 minutes.

To serve, place each packet on a plate, open the package and sprinkle with grated bottarga.

Note: Bottarga is the dried pressed roe of mullet or tuna and is available at speciality food stores. Alternatively, add 1 chopped anchovy to the mixture you pour over the fish.

I personally have cooked this recipe, and this is no exaggeration, at least one hundred thousand times in my life, especially after opening my second restaurant, a contemporary fine-dining establishment that specialized in seafood, at the age of twenty-two. This recipe is a favourite of mine because it combines glorious seafood, delicious coconut, and satisfying sweet potato. You can use pretty much any fish you wish with this dish, and it works just as well grilled, pan-roasted, or even poached in fish stock or the sauce as it does steamed. You can even make it with chicken, if seafood isn't your thing. To spice up the sauce a bit more, add additional chillies.

WILD SALMON
WITH COCONUT-LIME SAUCE & SWEET POTATO PUREE
SERVES 4

sweet potatoes
1¾ lb (800 g) sweet potatoes

1 tbsp peeled and grated
fresh ginger

1 tbsp coconut oil

coconut-lime sauce
1 tbsp coconut oil

2 tsp peeled and grated
fresh ginger

2 cloves garlic, finely chopped

1 red bird's eye chilli,
finely chopped

Finely grated zest of 1 lime

½ bunch of coriander stems,
chopped

2 lemongrass stalks, tender
white part only, finely chopped

2 kaffir lime leaves

2 cups (500 ml) coconut cream

1½ tbsp freshly squeezed
lime juice

1 tbsp fish sauce

1 tbsp raw honey

4 (6 oz/170 g) wild salmon fillets,
skin on, pin bones removed

2 tbsp fried shallots (page 207)

2 limes, peeled and segmented
(see page 209)

Fresh baby herbs, to garnish

Preheat the oven to 350°F (180°C gas 4). Bake the whole sweet potatoes for 1½ to 2 hours, or until tender.

Meanwhile, to make the coconut-lime sauce, heat the coconut oil in a pan over medium heat. Add the ginger, garlic, chilli, lime zest, coriander stems, and lemongrass and sauté until just starting to colour, about 1 minute. Tear the kaffir limes leaves, add to the pan with the coconut cream, and simmer for 30 minutes. Stir in the lime juice, fish sauce, and honey. Process in a blender and then pass through a fine-mesh sieve to remove any lumps.

To finish the sweet potatoes, pound the ginger in a mortar and pestle, then add ½ cup (125 ml) water. Leave to infuse for 30 minutes. Strain, reserving the ginger juice. Peel the skin off the baked sweet potatoes and puree the flesh with the ginger juice, coconut oil, and a bit of sea salt and white pepper. Keep warm.

To prepare the salmon, make a cut in the skin of each fillet, place in a steaming basket over simmering water, and steam for 6 minutes, or until the fish is just cooked through. (Add any extra aromatics you might have around to the simmering water, such as additional lemongrass or kaffir lime leaves, lemon, or star anise.) Transfer the fish to a plate, tent with foil, and let rest for 2 minutes.

Gently reheat the coconut-lime sauce, then pour into the middle of each of four plates, dividing it evenly. Place a mound of warm sweet potato puree on top and then top with a salmon fillet. Sprinkle the fried shallots, lime segments, and baby herbs around the fish and serve.

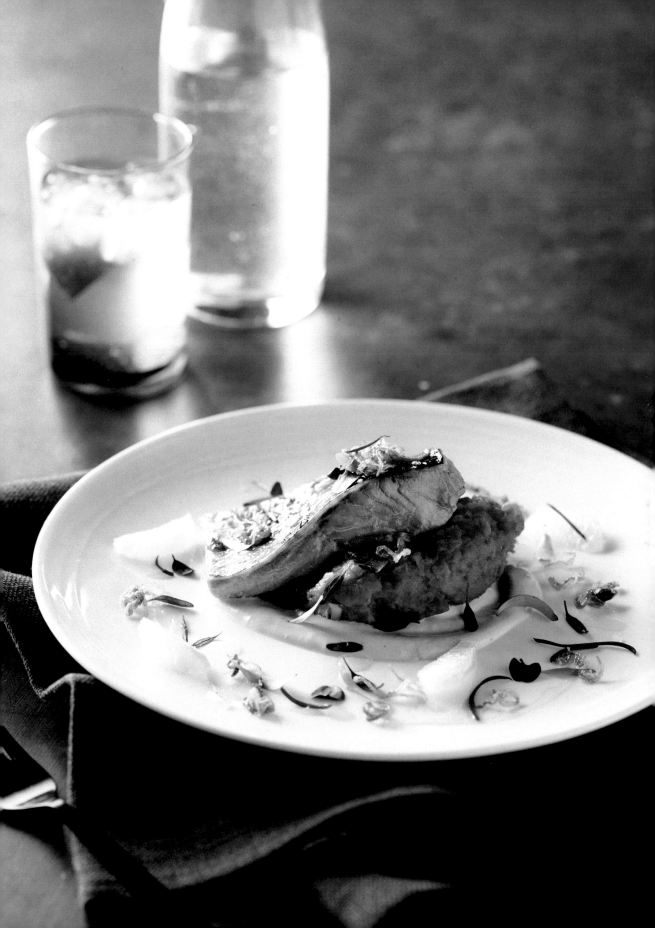

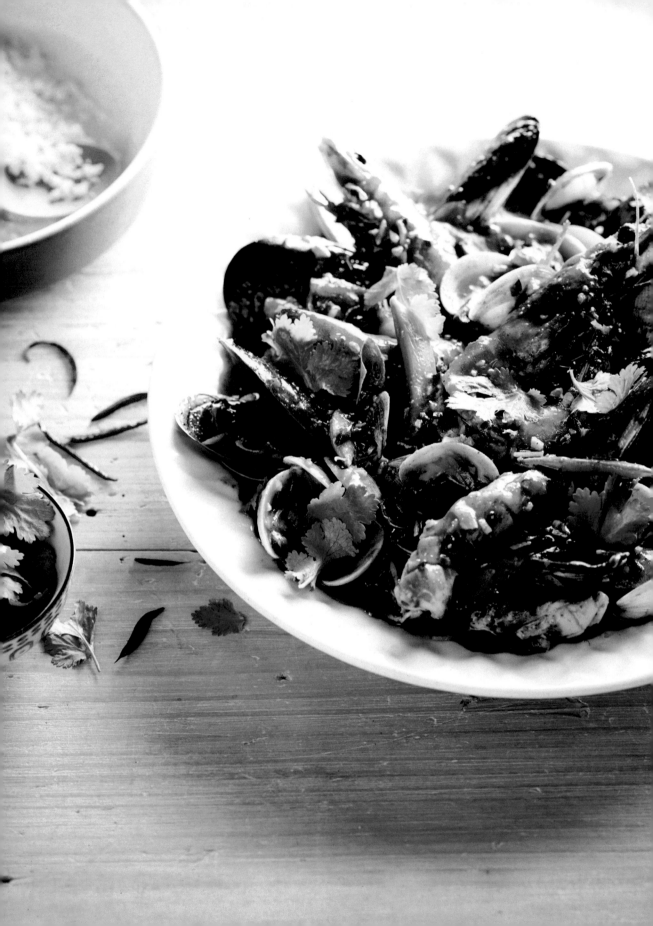

I spend a lot of time surfing and fishing, two activities that keep me energized and connected to nature. Sustainable fishing is something I am very passionate about, so much so that I am an ambassador for the World Wildlife Fund. The best thing we can do is to catch fish ourselves and not take more from the sea than is legal, so fisheries have a chance for survival. Additionally, look for sustainable sources of seafood. Buy locally if you can, and don't waste a mouthful. That is where a recipe like this – filled with prawns, squid, mussels, and clams – comes into play because you can use pretty much any type of seafood, and it will taste awesome.

SEAFOOD CURRY
SERVES 4

4 tbsp coconut oil

8 king prawns, peeled, tails intact, and de-veined

3½ oz (100 g) squid, cleaned and scored (page 208)

4 tbsp red curry paste (page 204)

1½ tsp tomato paste

2 vine-ripened tomatoes, chopped

1½ cups (375 ml) fish stock (page 202) or water

2 tbsp tamarind pulp

7 oz (200 g) clams, cleaned

7 oz (200 g) mussels, cleaned

3½ oz (100 g) sugar snap peas (optional)

4 aubergines, cut into ¾-inch (2 cm) pieces

1 tbsp peeled and grated fresh ginger

2 to 3 kaffir lime leaves, coarsely torn

2 tbsp fish sauce, plus more if needed

2 fresh red chillies, seeded and sliced

1 handful of fresh coriander leaves

Juice of 1 lime

Cauliflower Rice (page 61), to serve

Heat a large pan or wok over high heat. When hot, add 1 tbsp of the coconut oil and swirl around the wok. Add the prawns and squid in batches and cook until slightly golden and just cooked, 1 to 2 minutes. Remove from the wok and set aside.

Wipe the wok clean and add 1 tbsp of the coconut oil. Add the curry paste and tomato paste and allow it to cook until the paste separates from the oil and turns red and fragrant, 2 minutes. Stirring constantly, add the tomatoes and cook for 3 minutes, or until the tomatoes break down. Add the fish stock and tamarind pulp, bring to a boil, then reduce the heat to medium and simmer for 5 minutes, or until the sauce comes together. Add the clams, mussels, sugar snap peas (if using), aubergines, ginger, and kaffir lime leaves and toss together. Cover and cook for 3 to 4 minutes, until the clams and mussels open (discard any that do not open).

Return the squid and prawns to the wok, add the fish sauce, and toss and cook until heated through, about 1 minute. Remove from the heat and add the sliced chillies. Season with sea salt and freshly cracked black pepper, or add more fish sauce if it's needed. Finally, toss through the coriander and lime juice. Serve with the cauliflower rice.

This recipe is perfect for almost any type of fish. Sardines or even prawns and scallops are delectable prepared this way as well. I have, of course, ditched the wheat flour and breadcrumbs. You can either bake the fish in the oven at 350°F (175°C gas 3), or you can shallow-fry it until it's golden and crispy. My family loves to help coat the fish: I slice it, Indii dips it in the coconut flour, Nic dips it in the egg, and Chilli dips it in the crumb mix, and we always have a good laugh while we're doing it. Serve this with plenty of lemon, some artichoke tartar sauce (page 204), and a delicious simple green salad.

FISH & CHIPS

SERVES 4

1½ cups (200 g) macadamia nuts, activated (page 209) and chopped into fine crumbs or finely ground in a food processor

⅔ cup (50 g) unsweetened shredded dried coconut

2 tbsp chopped fresh flat-leaf parsley leaves

¾ cup (100 g) tapioca flour

3 eggs, lightly whisked

1⅓ lb (600 g) fish fillets, skins removed

Coconut oil, for shallow frying

Sweet Potato Fries with Rosemary and Sage (page 42)

Lemon wedges

Artichoke tartar sauce (page 204)

Mix together the macadamia crumbs, shredded coconut, and parsley in a bowl. Put the flour in a shallow bowl and the eggs in another bowl. Lightly season the fish with sea salt and freshly cracked black pepper, then dust lightly with the flour, coat in the egg, and roll in the crumbs, patting them on firmly.

Melt the oil in a frying pan over medium heat; it should be about 2 inches (5 cm) deep. When it reaches 320°F (160°C), shallow-fry the fish until golden and crispy on the first side, about 1 minute. Turn over and cook until crispy on the other side, about 1 minute more. Drain on paper towels and season with salt.

Serve with the sweet potato fries, lemon wedges, and tartar sauce.

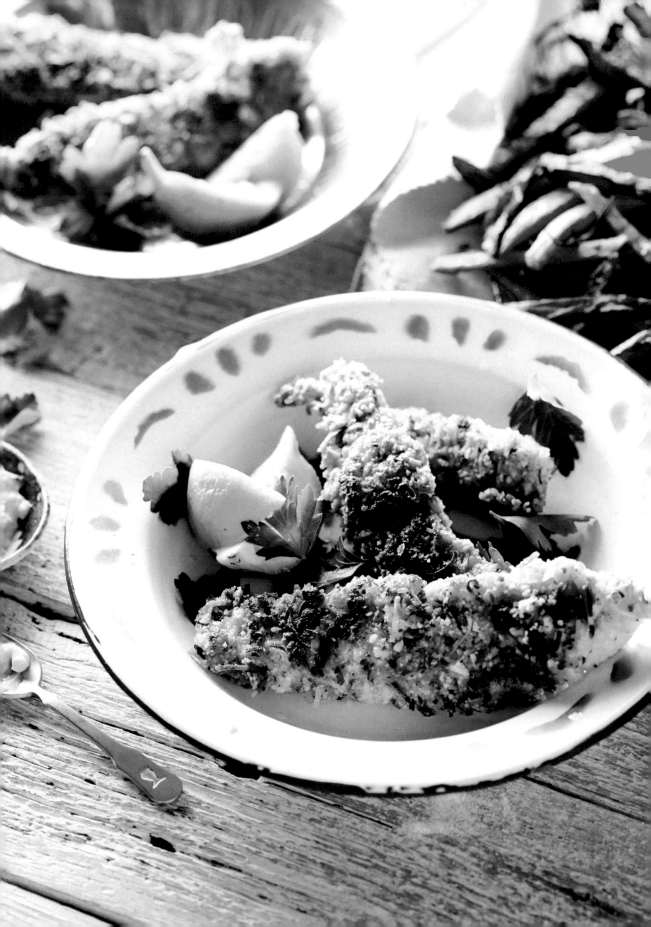

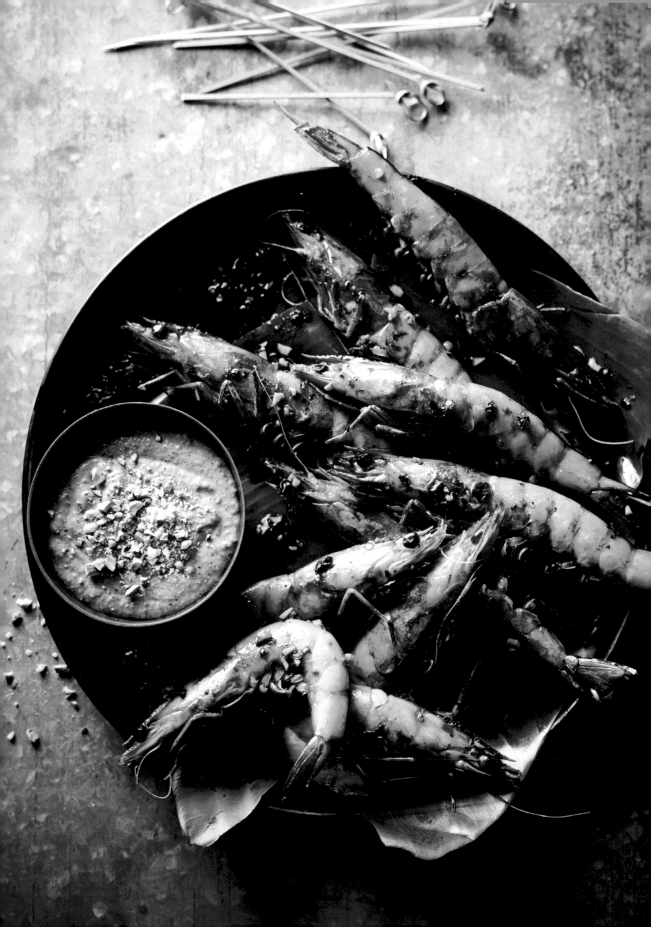

The smell of prawns cooking on the barbecue on a sunny summer afternoon may be one of the most intoxicating aromas I've ever known. The secret to cooking great prawns on a barbecue or over an open fire is to first remove the intestinal tract by inserting a skewer just below the head on the upper side of the prawn and carefully pulling it out, being careful not to break it. Cook the prawns with the head and shell on until lightly charred on the outside, ensuring that the flesh is still juicy and being careful not to overcook them. Cooking them this way is not only super easy, but it gets everyone involved with peeling them, which is a lot of fun. I personally eat them with the shell on and chew the heads, but feel free to peel them if you prefer. I won't judge!

PRAWN SATAY

SERVES 4

satay sauce
1 cup (140 g) raw cashews, activated (page 209)

½ cup (125 g) almond butter

2 tbsp peeled and grated fresh ginger

1 fresh red chilli, seeded and chopped

2 tbsp wheat-free tamari or coconut aminos

1 tbsp toasted sesame oil

1 tbsp maple syrup

prawn and marinade
4 cloves garlic, finely chopped

1-inch (2.5 cm) piece fresh ginger, peeled and grated

4 tbsp wheat-free tamari or coconut aminos

4 tbsp coconut oil, melted

1 tbsp red chilli flakes

1 tsp ground cumin

16 king prawns, head and tails intact

to serve
1 small handful of fresh coriander

1 fresh red chilli, chopped

1 lime, quartered

Soak sixteen bamboo skewers in water for 30 minutes.

To make the satay sauce, combine the cashews and almond butter in the bowl of a food processor and pulse until the nuts are fairly well ground. Add the ginger and fresh chilli. Processes until the mixture is well blended. Add the tamari, sesame oil, and maple syrup to the sauce. Blend well. With the motor running, pour in ¼ cup (60 ml) water and process until the sauce is smooth. Set aside in a bowl.

To make the marinade, combine the garlic, ginger, tamari, coconut oil, dried red chilli flakes, and cumin in a large bowl. Add the prawns and let marinate for 10 minutes. Thread the prawns onto the skewers through the tails straight up to the head.

Heat a barbecue or grill pan on high. Cook the prawns for 1½ to 2 minutes on each side, until they change colour and are cooked through. Season with sea salt and freshly cracked black pepper.

To serve, place the skewers on four serving plates or a platter. Garnish with the coriander and chilli and serve with lime wedges and the satay sauce.

POULTRY

112
vietnamese chicken wings

115
turkey & shiitake
lettuce cups

116
young coconut chicken salad

119
japanese crispy chicken
with miso mayonnaise

120
chicken salad with avocado
ranch dressing

123
jerk chicken with
papaya-mango salsa

124
hot & sour duck livers
with asian herb salad

127
chicken schnitzel with slaw

128
cauliflower fried rice
with chicken

131
grilled honey-mustard quail

132
robb wolf's quick
chicken curry

135
roast chicken thighs with
garlic, lemon & herbs

When I was a kid, my mother made chicken wings frequently, and I can still remember the smell that would radiate from her kitchen. I loved not only the gelatinous, moist texture of the meat, but also the sticky soy and honey sauce she used to glaze them. I have tried to stay true to my mum's original recipe here, but I have also added in a few more complex flavours that work wonderfully well. Of course, you can use this marinade and sauce on any part of the chicken, or even on duck, lamb, or pork for a flavour feast!

VIETNAMESE CHICKEN WINGS
SERVES 4

2 tbsp wheat-free tamari or coconut aminos

2 tbsp duck fat or coconut oil, melted

1 tbsp fish sauce

2 tsp raw honey (optional)

4 cloves garlic, finely chopped

2 spring onions, finely chopped

1 tsp red chilli flakes

½ tsp Chinese five-spice powder

12 whole chicken wings

to serve
Fried shallots (page 207)

Fried chillies (page 207)

1 small handful of mixed fresh Asian herbs (Thai basil, coriander, Vietnamese mint)

Preheat the oven to 400°F (200°C gas 6).

To make the marinade, combine the tamari, duck fat, fish sauce, honey (if using), garlic, spring onions, red chilli flakes, and five-spice powder in a large mixing bowl and whisk together. Add the chicken wings and turn until the chicken is well coated. Cover and refrigerate for at least 1 hour or ideally overnight.

Transfer the wings to a baking sheet, spread into an even layer, and bake for 25 to 30 minutes, turning occasionally, until the chicken is golden and cooked through.

Arrange on a serving platter and sprinkle with the fried shallots, fried chillies, and Asian herbs.

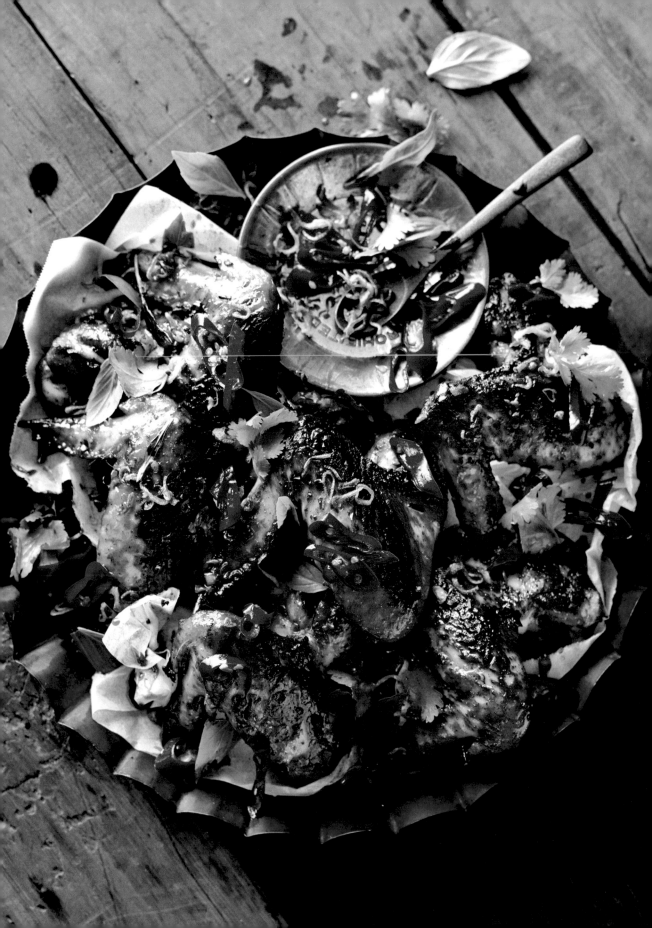

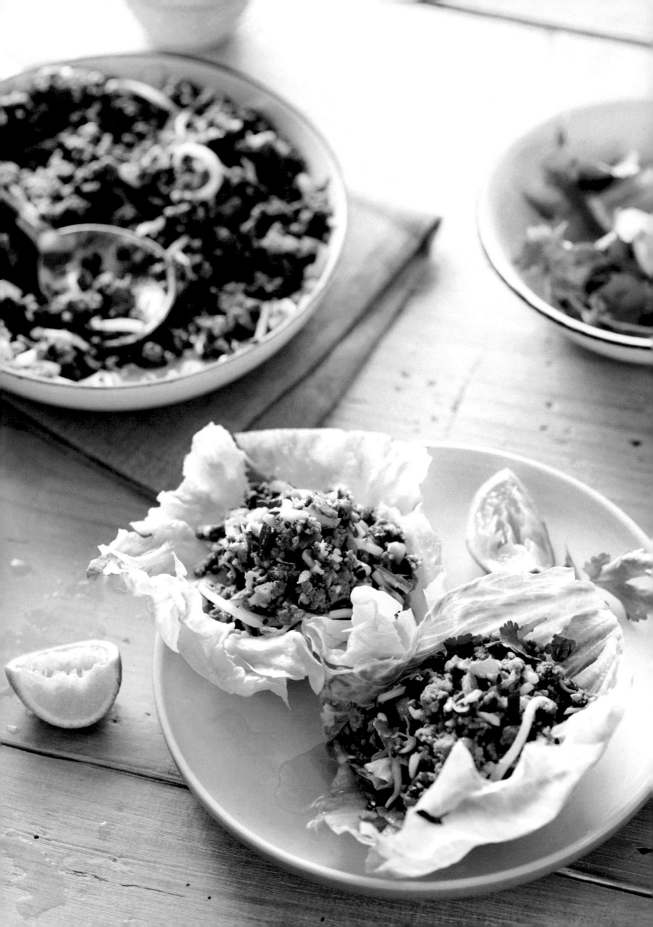

I just adore these salad cups because they are so versatile, and you can put all kinds of things in them, including last night's leftovers. Once you have your protein and salad ingredients, just toss them with your favourite salad dressing or sauce – whether dairy-free pesto, tahini, salsa verde, aïoli (page 203) flavoured with horseradish, or even roasted garlic and lemon. Here, I've used an Asian-style preparation to add a bit of kick. This is extremely popular with ravenous teenagers as a healthy lunchtime feast after doing weekend sports!

TURKEY & SHIITAKE LETTUCE CUPS
SERVES 4

1 tbsp coconut oil, ghee, or duck fat

3 cloves garlic, finely chopped

4 shallots, chopped

2 tsp peeled and grated fresh ginger

1⅓ lb (600 g) minced turkey

4 oz (120 g) shiitake mushrooms, chopped

2 tbsp wheat-free tamari or coconut aminos

1 tbsp fish sauce, plus more to serve

1 tsp raw honey (optional)

1 (8 oz/225 g) can water chestnuts, drained and finely chopped

4 spring onions, finely chopped

2 fresh red chillies, seeded and chopped

3½ oz (100 g) bean sprouts

8 iceberg lettuce leaves, washed and dried

Fresh coriander leaves, torn, to serve

Lime wedges, to serve

Heat a wok or large frying pan over medium-high heat. When hot, add the coconut oil and swirl around the wok. Add the garlic, shallots, and ginger and cook for 1 minute. Add the turkey and mushrooms and cook for another 4 to 5 minutes, stirring occasionally, until cooked through and browned. Add the tamari, fish sauce, and honey, if using, and toss to mix. Then add the water chestnuts, spring onions, and chillies and keep stirring until the mixture is well combined. Cook until heated through, 2 to 3 minutes. Remove from the heat, mix in the bean sprouts, and check for seasoning, adding more fish sauce or sea salt if needed.

To serve, place the lettuce cups on a serving platter or four plates. Top each with some of the turkey mixture, and garnish with coriander leaves and lime wedges.

Young coconuts are awesome, from the sweet, energizing water contained in the nut itself to the young jelly-like flesh. Revered for its health benefits, the flesh is extremely versatile; you can blend it into a creamy salad dressing, use it for desserts or snacks, thicken smoothies with it, or add it to curries or stir-fries. My favourite way to enjoy young coconuts is to serve a Vietnamese-inspired salad in half of one – just eat the coconut as you eat the salad. Or you can remove the flesh, shred it, and add it directly to the salad. Either way is great!

YOUNG COCONUT CHICKEN SALAD
SERVES 4

pickled onion
½ red onion, thinly sliced

3 tbsp raw apple cider vinegar

fish sauce dressing
⅓ cup (80 ml) fish sauce

2 tbsp peeled and grated fresh ginger

3 cloves garlic, finely chopped

1 to 2 fresh red chillies, finely chopped

3 to 4 tbsp lime juice, or to taste

1 tbsp raw honey (optional)

chicken
1 lb (500 g) boneless, skinless chicken thighs

3⅓ cups (830 ml) coconut milk

2 tbsp fish sauce

1 tbsp peeled and grated fresh ginger

1 clove garlic, finely chopped

salad
4¼ cups (300 g) thinly shredded cabbage

2 handfuls of fresh coriander leaves

1 handful of fresh mint leaves

1 handful of fresh Thai or holy basil leaves

½ cup (80 g) shredded carrot

to serve
2 young green coconuts

3 tbsp fried shallots (page 207)

2 tbsp fried garlic (page 207)

3 oz (80 g) almonds, activated (page 209), roasted, and crushed

To pickle the onion, combine the onion and vinegar in a bowl and let sit for 20 minutes, then drain. To make the fish sauce dressing, in a bowl or large jar, combine the fish sauce, ⅓ cup (80 ml) water, ginger, garlic, chillies, lime juice, and honey, if using. Set aside.

To cook the chicken, place the chicken thighs in a pan and add the coconut milk, 1 cup (250 ml) water, the fish sauce, ginger, and garlic. Bring to a simmer over medium heat and cook until the chicken is cooked through, 10 to 12 minutes. Set aside to cool. Once the chicken is cool enough to handle, shred the meat.

To make the salad, in a large bowl, combine the cabbage, coriander, mint, basil, and carrot and toss well.

To prepare the coconut bowls, using a large, sharp, heavy knife, cut each coconut in half around the middle. Pour out the water and reserve it for another use. Using a large kitchen spoon, gently run the spoon between the flesh and the peel in a circular motion around the coconut while trying not to break the flesh. Carefully slide the spoon underneath to the bottom and lift the coconut flesh out.

When you're ready to serve, toss the chicken into the salad and add the fish sauce dressing to taste. Top with the fried shallots, fried garlic, almonds, and pickled onion.

Divide the salad between the four coconut bowls, scooping out the young coconut flesh as you eat the salad.

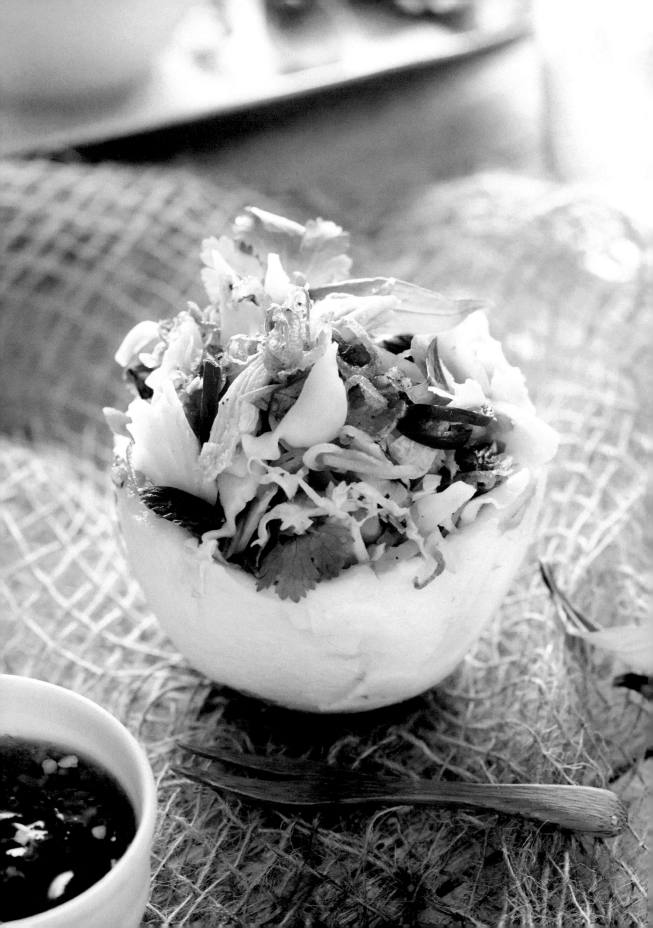

Note: If you like, soak bamboo skewers in water
for 30 minutes, then thread the marinated
chicken on the skewers, coat with ground almonds,
and fry the chicken on the skewers.

One of my favourite foods is fried chicken, so I needed to find a Paleo alternative to the classic version. I have managed to come up with many recipes that keep me happy, but none more so than this Japanese-inspired version. I love serving it with a really fresh and crispy mooli (Japanese white radish) salad or even just a lovely spring onion salad that packs a punch. But don't stop here; play around with different spices and herbs and take inspiration from around the globe.

JAPANESE CRISPY CHICKEN
WITH MISO MAYONNAISE
SERVES 4

miso mayonnaise
½ cup (120 ml) mayonnaise (page 203)

1 tsp white miso paste

1 tbsp bonito flakes, crushed in your hands to form a powder

marinade & chicken
1 tsp peeled and grated fresh ginger

2 cloves garlic, finely chopped

1 egg yolk

2 tbsp white wine

3 tbsp wheat-free tamari or coconut aminos

1 tbsp toasted sesame oil

1¾ lb (800 g) boneless, skinless chicken thighs, cut into 2-inch (5 cm) pieces

¾ cup (75 g) ground almonds

¾ cup (90 g) tapioca starch

Coconut oil, for frying

to serve
Fresh baby shiso leaves

Black and white sesame seeds, toasted

Ichimi togarashi (Japanese ground red chilli; optional)

To make the miso mayonnaise, combine the mayonnaise, miso, and bonito powder and mix until blended. Set aside.

To make the marinade, combine the ginger, garlic, egg yolk, wine, tamari, sesame oil, 1 tsp sea salt, and some freshly cracked black pepper. Add the chicken, turning the pieces until well coated. Marinate in the refrigerator for 10 to 15 minutes.

In a shallow bowl, mix together the ground almonds and tapioca starch. Lift the chicken out of the marinade and coat the chicken with the ground almond mixture, shaking off any excess.

Fill a wok or saucepan halfway with coconut oil and heat over medium heat to 340°F (170°C). Add one piece of chicken to the oil to test; it should bubble right away. Deep-fry the chicken in batches until golden brown, crispy and cooked through, 2 to 3 minutes. Place on paper towels to drain the excess oil. Season with salt and pepper.

To serve, thread the chicken pieces onto eight skewers. Garnish with the shiso leaves, sesame seeds, and *ichimi togarashi*. Pass the mayonnaise alongside.

What is it about chicken salad that everyone loves? I remember at my first restaurant we offered a modest grilled chicken Caesar salad and sold more of those than any other item! The wonderful thing about salads is that you do not need to fill it up with protein; a 2- to 3-ounce (50 to 75 g) portion per person is more than satisfying. Just make sure the bulk of the salad includes fresh lettuce, vegetables, nuts, seeds, an amazing dressing, and perhaps some fruit. My trick is to cook extra chicken when making it for another recipe. The extra meat can be shredded or chopped and put into whatever concoctions my imagination can create.

CHICKEN SALAD
WITH AVOCADO RANCH DRESSING
SERVES 4 TO 6

avocado ranch dressing

1 ripe avocado, peeled, pitted and mashed

2 tbsp extra virgin olive oil

2 tbsp coconut cream

1 tbsp raw apple cider vinegar

1 tbsp each chopped fresh flat-leaf parsley and dill

1 tsp fermented mustard (page 206)

½ tsp onion powder

2 boneless chicken breasts

2 tbsp ghee, duck fat, or coconut oil, melted

salad

4 celery hearts with leaves, chopped

2 Granny Smith apples, cored and thinly sliced

2 heads chicory, leaves separated and torn

1 large handful each of frisée and lamb's lettuce leaves

½ bunch of tarragon leaves, torn

⅓ cup (40 g) raisins

⅓ cup (30 g) walnuts, activated (page 209), toasted, and coarsely chopped

⅓ cup (80 ml) good-quality extra virgin olive oil

2 tbsp raw apple cider vinegar

To make the ranch dressing, combine the avocado, 4 tbsp water, oil, coconut cream, vinegar, parsley, dill, mustard, and onion powder in a food processor and process until smooth. Season with sea salt and freshly cracked black pepper to taste. Transfer the dressing to a bowl, cover, and place in the refrigerator until needed.

Preheat the oven to 400°F (200°C gas 6). Rub the chicken with some of the ghee and season with salt and pepper. Heat a large frying pan with the remaining ghee and sear the chicken, skin side down, until crisp and lightly golden, 2 minutes. Turn over the chicken and sear the other side until lightly golden, 1 minute. Place the chicken on a baking sheet and roast, skin side up, for 7 minutes, or until cooked through. Remove from the oven and allow to cool.

Remove the crispy skin from the chicken and slice the skin into small strips. Slice the flesh into ⅓-inch (1 cm) slices and set aside.

To make the salad, combine the celery, apples, chicory, frisée, lamb's lettuce, tarragon, raisins, and walnuts in a bowl. Mix together the oil and vinegar and drizzle over the salad. Add the chicken slices and crispy skin strips and season with salt and pepper. Toss to combine.

To serve, transfer the salad to a serving platter or bowl and drizzle over some of the avocado ranch dressing. Pass the remaining dressing on the side.

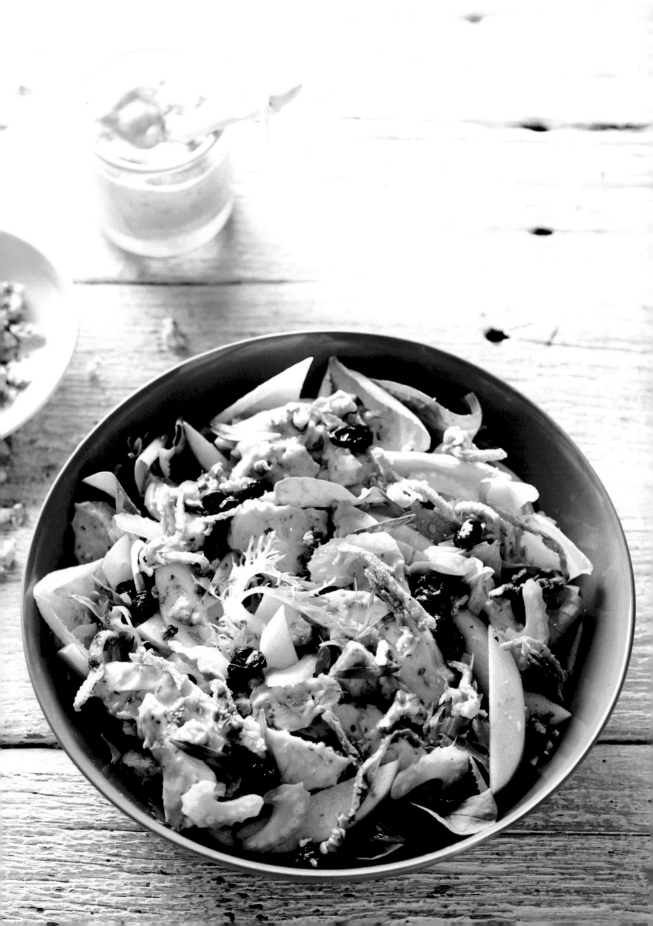

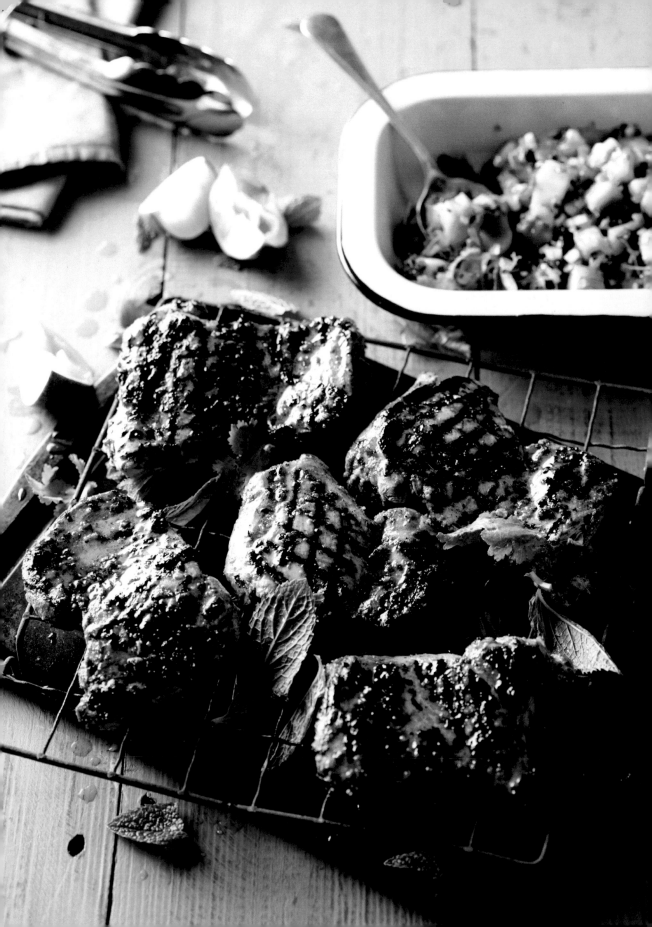

Jerk is a Jamaican marinade that is tremendous when partnered with a variety of meats, including chicken, pork, lamb, and seafood, or even eggs. Jerk seasonings can differ, but the main flavours are allspice and chilli, with the following added in whatever ratios or combinations the cook feels like: cloves, cinnamon, spring onions, garlic, nutmeg, thyme, salt, and pepper. I use chicken thighs or legs when I am cooking this recipe because I find the fat content keeps the chicken juicy and allows the meat to hold a lot more flavour than the breast. But do not be afraid to rub jerk seasoning all over a whole chicken or duck and roast it in the oven for an extraordinary culinary delicacy.

JERK CHICKEN
WITH PAPAYA-MANGO SALSA
SERVES 4

jerk chicken
1 red onion, chopped

3 spring onions, chopped

6 cloves garlic, finely chopped

4 habanero chillies, seeded

¼ cup (60 ml) freshly squeezed lime juice

3 tbsp wheat-free tamari or coconut aminos

3 tbsp coconut oil, melted

1 tbsp white wine vinegar

1 tbsp raw honey (optional)

1 tbsp fresh thyme leaves

1 tbsp smoked paprika

2 tsp ground allspice

½ tsp ground cinnamon

¼ tsp freshly grated nutmeg

2 bay leaves

2¼ lb (1 kg) boneless chicken thighs, with skin

papaya-mango salsa
½ papaya, peeled, seeded, and diced into ⅓-inch (1 cm) cubes

1 mango, peeled and diced into ⅓-inch (1 cm) cubes

½ red onion, finely chopped

1 jalapeño chilli, seeded and finely chopped

1 fresh red chilli, finely chopped

3 tbsp freshly squeezed lime juice

2 tbsp chopped fresh coriander leaves, plus more to serve

2 tbsp chopped fresh mint leaves, plus more to serve

Lime wedges, to serve

To make the chicken, combine the red onion, spring onions, garlic, habaneros, lime juice, tamari, coconut oil, white wine vinegar, honey, if using, thyme, paprika, allspice, cinnamon, nutmeg, 2 tsp freshly cracked black pepper, and 1½ tsp sea salt in a food processor. Process to form a smooth paste. Transfer to a large shallow dish, add the bay leaves and chicken, and turn to coat the chicken. Cover and refrigerate overnight for best results.

To make the papaya-mango salsa, combine the papaya, mango, red onion, jalapeño, red chilli, lime juice, coriander, and mint in a bowl. Mix gently together, season with a little salt, and set aside.

Bring the chicken to room temperature before cooking. Preheat a barbecue or grill pan to medium-high heat. Remove the chicken from the marinade. Grill, turning and basting occasionally with the marinade for 15 minutes, or until the chicken is cooked through. Cover with foil and allow it to rest for 5 to 10 minutes.

To serve, arrange the chicken on a platter with the lime wedges and sprinkle over some coriander and mint leaves. Pass the salsa on the side.

Liver is one of the most important parts of the animal to eat because, generally, organ meats are between ten to one hundred times higher in nutrients than corresponding muscle meats. In ancient cultures, they were revered so much that the organs were eaten first, and the muscle meats were the last to be eaten. Today, liver is probably the most widely eaten organ meat in the West, and the one that most people have tried, commonly in a pâté. This recipe is a lovely way to enjoy liver in a different way. It is heavily flavoured with a spiced dressing and served with lots of aromatic herbs that will keep you coming back for more and more and more.

HOT & SOUR DUCK LIVERS
WITH ASIAN HERB SALAD
SERVES 4

dressing
½ cup (120 ml) freshly squeezed lime juice

2 tbsp fish sauce

½ tsp toasted sesame oil

2 tbsp raw honey (optional)

1 to 2 tsp red chilli flakes

1 clove garlic, finely chopped

duck livers
1⅓ lb (600 g) duck or chicken livers, sinews and fat removed

3 tbsp coconut oil or duck fat

herb salad
½ bunch of mint leaves, torn

1 bunch of Vietnamese mint leaves, torn

1 bunch of coriander leaves, torn

1 bunch of Thai basil leaves, torn

3 fresh red chillies, seeded and sliced

3 spring onions, green parts only, thinly sliced

2 kaffir lime leaves, finely julienned

1 tsp white sesame seeds

3 small heirloom tomatoes, preferably green zebra, thinly sliced

1 cucumber, thinly sliced lengthwise into long strips

Sunflower seeds, activated (page 209), to serve

To make the dressing, in a bowl, whisk together the lime juice, fish sauce, sesame oil, honey, if using, chilli flakes, and garlic; set aside.

To prepare the livers, season with sea salt and freshly cracked black pepper and set aside. Add the coconut oil to a large frying pan or a wok over medium heat and allow it to heat for 30 seconds. Place the livers in the pan in a single layer, in two batches if necessary. Cook until browned on one side, about 2 minutes, then turn and cook until browned on the other side, 1 to 2 minutes more. Transfer to a plate and let rest for 3 minutes. They should be pink in the centre.

To make the herb salad, in a large bowl, combine the mint, Vietnamese mint, coriander, Thai basil, chillies, spring onions, lime leaves, sesame seeds, tomatoes, and cucumber. Add the livers and carefully toss.

Transfer the salad to a platter and drizzle with a good amount of the dressing. Sprinkle with the sunflower seeds. Serve, passing any extra dressing on the side.

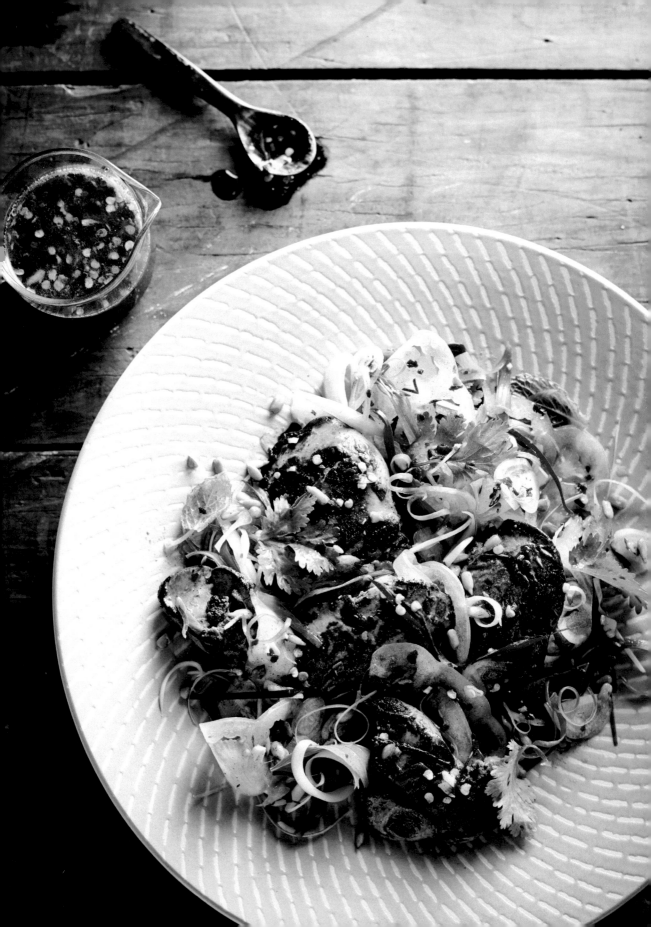

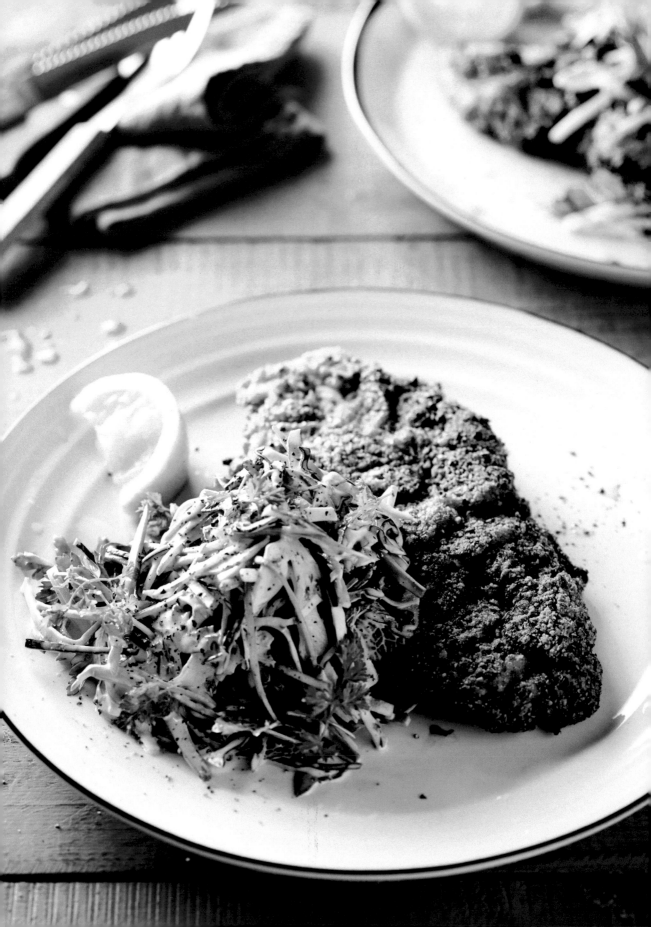

The first word that springs to my mind whenever I hear the word *schnitzel* is 'yum'. I have loved schnitzel ever since I was young boy, and I reckon I will love it until I am old. Originally from Austria, schnitzel is thinly sliced meat, most classically veal, tenderized until it is flat and uniform in thickness. It is then dusted in seasoned flour, dipped in egg, dredged in breadcrumbs, and pan-fried until golden and crispy. This Paleo version is equally tasty. I've chosen to make it with chicken; tapioca flour is used to lightly dust the meat, which is then dredged through eggs and coated in seasoned ground almonds.

CHICKEN SCHNITZEL
WITH SLAW
SERVES 2

2 boneless, skinless chicken thighs or breasts, sinew and veins removed (about 12 oz/340 g)

10 oz (300 g) ground almonds, plus more if needed

2 tsp garlic powder

2 tsp onion powder

1 tsp chilli powder, such as ancho

2 tsp dried parsley

⅓ cup (60 g) tapioca flour

3 eggs

⅓ cup (80 ml) coconut milk

About 2 cups (500 ml) coconut oil, for shallow frying

Root Vegetable Slaw with Chervil Mayonnaise (page 58)

Lemon wedges, to serve

Between two sheets of waxed paper, bash your chicken until it's about ¼ inch (5 mm) thick.

Combine the ground almonds with the garlic powder, onion powder, chilli powder, and dried parsley in a bowl and mix well. Season with sea salt and freshly cracked black pepper and set aside.

Dust the chicken with the tapioca flour, shake off any excess, and set aside.

Whisk the eggs and coconut milk in another bowl until well combined.

Drop the chicken (one at a time) in the egg mixture and turn so it is completely coated. Then place the chicken in the ground almond mixture and turn to coat evenly on both sides.

Heat a frying pan over a medium-high heat with the coconut oil; it should come to a depth of about 1½ inches (4 cm). When the oil reaches 325°F (160°C), add the chicken and fry on both sides until golden and cooked through, 3 to 5 minutes. Remove from the pan and place on paper towels to soak up the excess oil. Season with salt and pepper.

Serve the chicken schnitzels with the slaw and lemon wedges.

The more I make this recipe, the more I love it; actually, the more I eat this recipe, the more I love cooking it! Cauliflower fried rice is seriously delicious and it takes less than ten minutes to get a load of it on the table. I love playing around with ingredients in this recipe by adding different spices and herbs; proteins like prawns, crab, turkey, ham, or nitrate-free bacon; and an assortment of veggies to create a deliciously balanced meal. If it's hot outside and you want to make a cool, refreshing dish, just let this cool down or chill it in the fridge and add it to any salad.

CAULIFLOWER FRIED RICE
WITH CHICKEN

SERVES 4

1 head cauliflower, separated into florets

2 tbsp coconut oil

4 slices bacon or ham, finely diced

1 lb (450 g) boneless, skinless chicken thighs, cut into 1-inch (2.5 cm) pieces

4 eggs, whisked with a splash of fish sauce to season

1 brown onion, finely chopped

2 cloves garlic, finely chopped

½ red pepper, seeded and diced

1-inch (2.5 cm) piece fresh ginger, peeled and grated

1 cup (100 g) sliced okra

1¼ cups (100 g) sliced brussels sprouts

3 tbsp wheat-free tamari or coconut aminos

2 spring onions, thinly sliced

2 tbsp chopped fresh coriander leaves

2 tbsp chopped fresh flat-leaf parsley leaves

½ cup (50 g) bean sprouts

Fish sauce, to serve

Pulse the cauliflower in a food processor until its texture resembles rice.

In a large wok or frying pan, heat a little of the coconut oil over high heat. Add the bacon and fry until crispy, 2 to 3 minutes, then remove and set aside. Wipe out the wok and add a little more coconut oil. Add the chicken and sauté over high heat until golden and cooked through, about 3 minutes. Remove from the pan and set aside.

Wipe the wok clean again, turn down the heat to medium, and add a little more coconut oil. Pour the eggs into the pan and cook, tilting the wok to let the uncooked eggs slide underneath the set eggs. Flip the omelette and cook until slightly golden, about 2 minutes. Remove, slice into thin strips, and set aside.

Heat a little of the coconut oil in the wok over high heat, add the onion and garlic and cook until softened, about 3 minutes. Stir in the red pepper and ginger and cook until softened, 3 to 5 minutes. Add the okra and brussels sprouts and cook for 1 minute, then add the cauliflower and cook until tender, 2 to 3 minutes. Add the tamari, spring onions, coriander, parsley, bean sprouts, the reserved bacon, chicken, omelette strips, and sea salt and ground white pepper to taste, and stir-fry for 1 minute until well combined. Season with a splash of fish sauce, transfer to a serving bowl, and serve.

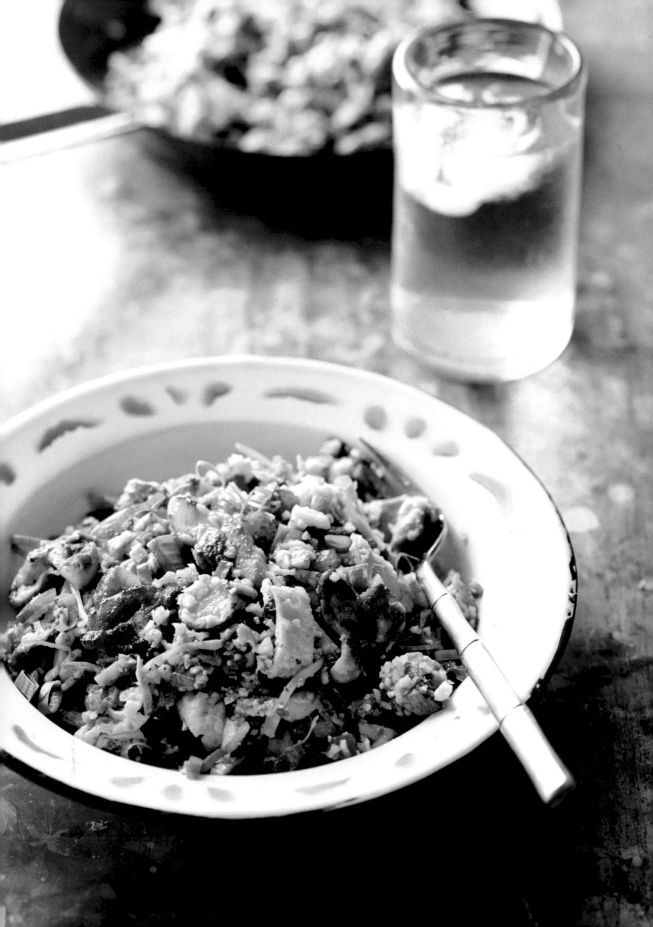

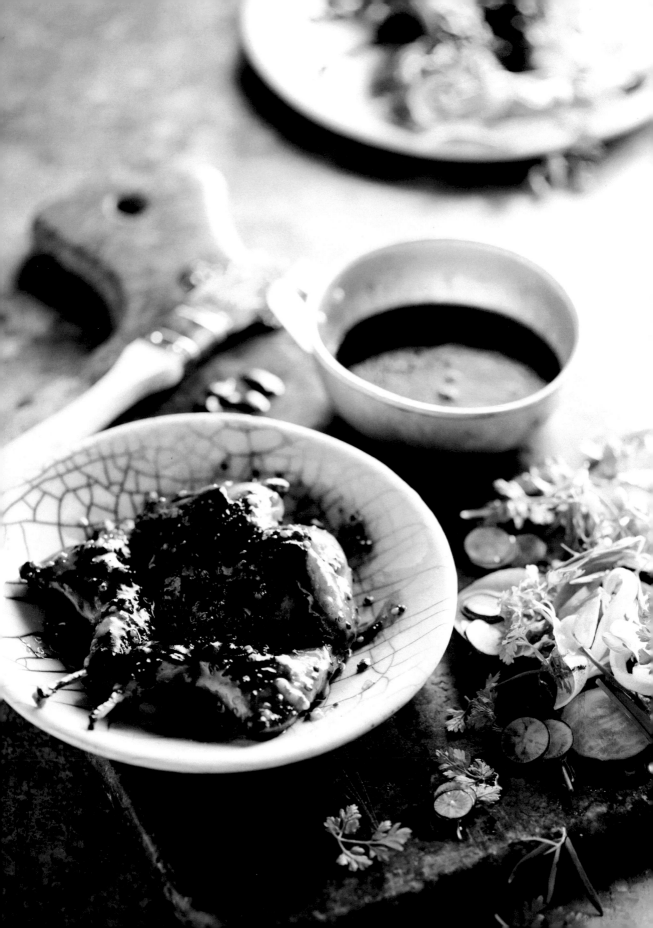

Quail has featured on my menus over the last few decades in different guises, and it's always been a hit. The key to cooking quail is all in the timing; you mustn't overcook it. The leg meat should be just falling off the bone and the breast meat should be tender, moist, and slightly pink. This honey-mustard marinade becomes lovely and golden when cooked and the flavours are a perfect accompaniment to the delicate game-like qualities of quail meat. If quail doesn't sound appealing to you, this marinade also works well with chicken, duck, and even pork.

GRILLED HONEY-MUSTARD QUAIL
SERVES 2

quail and marinade
4 tbsp raw honey

3 tbsp macadamia nut oil
or melted coconut oil

3 tbsp fermented mustard
(page 206)

3 tbsp balsamic vinegar

1 tbsp chopped fresh thyme

2 cloves garlic, finely chopped

2 whole quail, butterflied

herb salad
¼ bunch of chives, cut into
1-inch (2.5 cm) lengths

1 bunch of tarragon, torn

½ bunch of oregano leaves, torn

1 handful of fresh chervil leaves,
torn

1 fennel bulb, shaved

3 red radishes, thinly sliced

4 tbsp extra virgin olive oil

1 tbsp freshly squeezed
lemon juice

To make the marinade, combine the honey, macadamia nut oil, mustard, vinegar, thyme, and garlic in a bowl and mix well. Set aside ⅓ cup (80 ml) of the marinade and place in a separate container; refrigerate until ready to use. Add the quail to the remaining marinade and turn to coat. Marinate in the fridge for at least 1 hour, or for best results, overnight. Place the quail on a plate and season with sea salt and freshly cracked black pepper.

Preheat the oven to 400°F (200°C gas 6).

Preheat a grill pan or barbecue to high. Grill the quail for 2 minutes, skin side down, basting occasionally with the marinade. Turn and grill for 1 minute on the other side. Transfer the quail to a roasting tin and roast in the hot oven for 5 to 6 minutes, or until cooked through. Allow to rest for 2 to 3 minutes, keeping warm.

Heat the reserved ⅓ cup (80 ml) marinade in a small saucepan over medium heat and bring to a simmer. Remove the sauce from the heat and season with a touch of salt.

Just before you are ready to serve, make the herb salad. Mix together the chives, tarragon, oregano, chervil, fennel, and radishes in a bowl. Dress the salad with the olive oil and lemon juice. Arrange the salad on two serving plates, place the quail on top, spoon over the warm sauce, and serve.

Robb Wolf is a biochemist, the well-known author of *The Paleo Solution*, and one of the leading authorities on the Paleo diet. Robb has kindly shared one of his quick, easy, and delicious recipes for us to try, and it is a winner. Robb suggests that if you are in a hurry, use a pre-made curry paste, but always look for ones that do not contain sugar or trans fats. If you do have the time, I recommend that you make your own curry paste from scratch. And while you are at it, make a double or triple batch and freeze it in ice cube trays, then store it in the freezer and just pop one out whenever you want to whip up this dish. Serve this with Cauliflower Rice (page 61) and a big bowl of Asian greens or a large cucumber salad to meet all your nutritional needs.

ROBB WOLF'S QUICK CHICKEN CURRY
SERVES 4

2 tbsp coconut oil

1 brown onion, chopped

1⅓ lb (600 g) boneless, skinless chicken thighs, diced into 1-inch (2.5 cm) pieces

5 tbsp yellow curry paste (page 205)

16 whole okra pods

1 or 2 fresh red chillies, sliced

4 tbsp cashews, activated (page 209)

1⅔ cups (400 ml) coconut cream

2 tbsp fish sauce, plus more if needed

2 handfuls of fresh baby spinach

Handful of fresh coriander leaves

Lime wedges, to serve

Cauliflower Rice (page 61) or kelp noodles, to serve

Heat a wok over medium heat, then add the coconut oil and swirl around. Add the onion and sauté until translucent, 3 to 4 minutes. Increase the heat to high, add the chicken and sauté until the chicken is slightly coloured, 2 to 3 minutes. Add the curry paste and cook until fragrant, 1 minute. Add the okra, chilli, and cashews; give it a good toss; then pour in the coconut cream. Stir together then simmer for 5 minutes, or until the curry paste is nicely infused through the sauce and the sauce thickens slightly. Stir in the fish sauce, taste, and add more if you like. Remove from the heat, and stir in the spinach and coriander.

Transfer to a serving bowl and serve with lime wedges and cauliflower rice or kelp noodles.

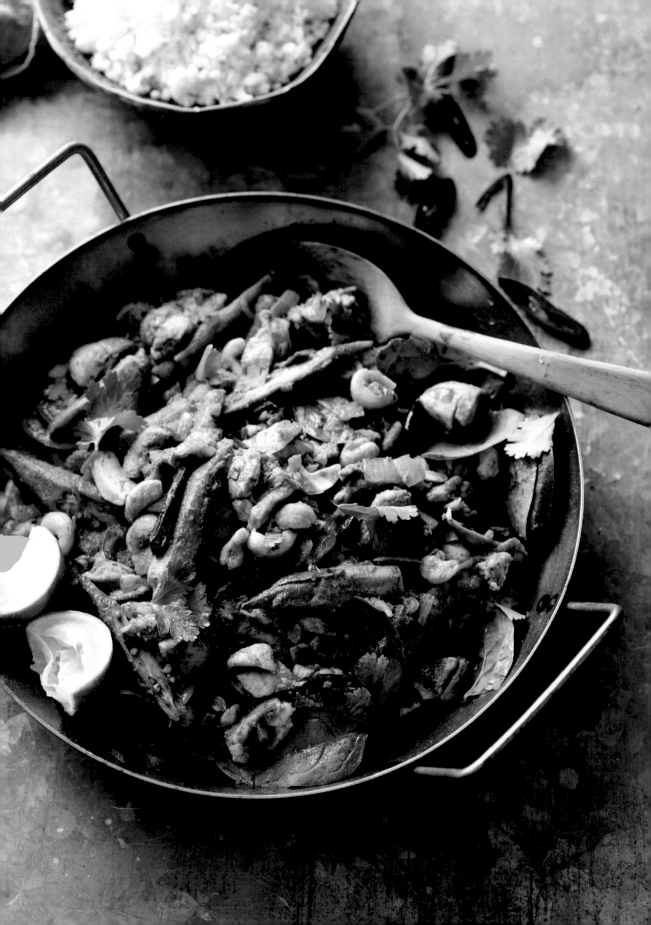

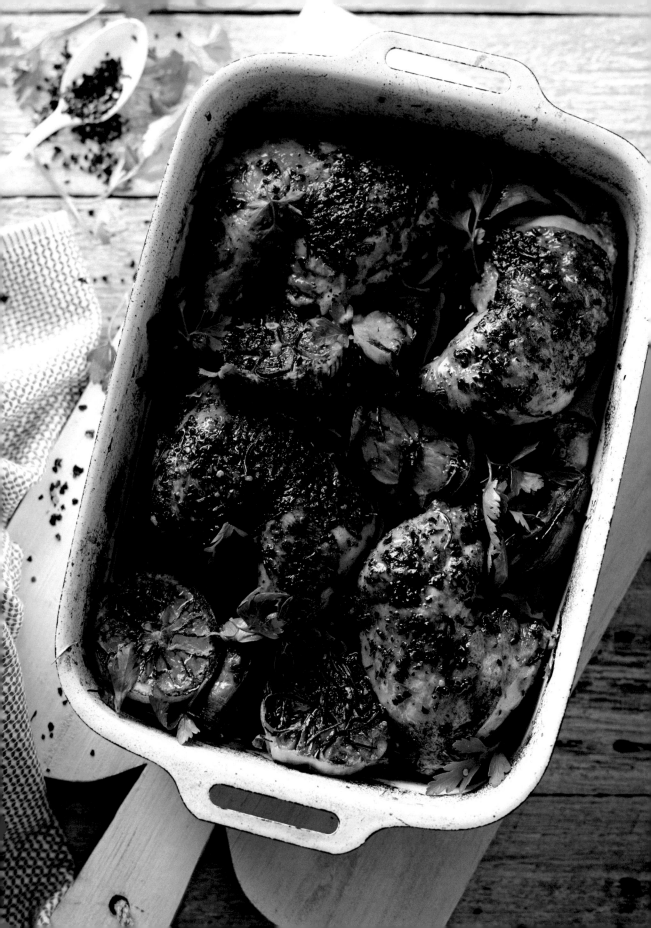

One of my goals is to write the roast chicken bible, describing all the different ways to roast chicken, not only because I would get to taste every single version, but because I think roast chicken is the most comforting, memory-invoking dish. The recipe here is a basic, yet flavour-filled, version of a gorgeous dish my Italian friend Marina has cooked for me a few times. I especially like it when the lemons get a bit burnt in the pan and the juices mix with the chicken fat, garlic, chilli, and rosemary to form the most delicious sauce known. *Bellissimo*!

ROAST CHICKEN THIGHS
WITH GARLIC, LEMON & HERBS
SERVES 4 TO 6

⅓ cup (80 g) duck fat, coconut oil, or ghee, melted

2 tbsp raw honey (optional)

1 tbsp dried Italian seasoning

1 tsp paprika

1 tsp onion powder

¼ tsp red chilli flakes

6 boneless, skin-on chicken thighs

3 lemons, halved or quartered

4 shallots, halved

2 heads garlic, halved

3 sprigs rosemary, chopped

1 tsp dried oregano

Chopped fresh herbs (such as rosemary, thyme, and/or parsley), for garnish

In a small bowl, whisk together the melted duck fat, honey, Italian seasoning, paprika, onion powder, red chilli flakes, and some sea salt and freshly cracked black pepper.

Place the chicken thighs in a 9 by 13-inch (23 by 33 cm) baking dish, skin side up. Pour the seasoning mixture all over the chicken, turning the pieces to coat all sides. Arrange the lemon pieces, shallots, and garlic around and under the chicken and sprinkle with the rosemary and oregano. For the best results, cover the chicken and marinate overnight in the refrigerator.

Preheat the oven to 400°F (200°C gas 6).

Season the chicken with salt and pepper. Roast, uncovered, for about 30 minutes, or until the chicken is cooked, the skin is crispy, and the juices run clear. Garnish with additional chopped fresh herbs, if desired.

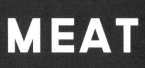

MEAT

139

mum's burgers

140

lamb meatballs with roasted
pumpkin, pomegranate
& tahini sauce

143

steak tartare

144

pork cutlets with cabbage
salad & romesco sauce

147

meatballs in chipotle sauce

148

grilled sirloin with
tomato-herb salad

151

venison skewers with
beetroot chimichurri

152

nom nom paleo's
surf & turf tacos

155

grilled sirloin with
mushrooms, horseradish
& rocket

156

portuguese pork burgers
with piri piri sauce

159

lamb liver kebabs with
sumac & parsley salad

160

seared beef liver with fig
salad & sherry vinaigrette

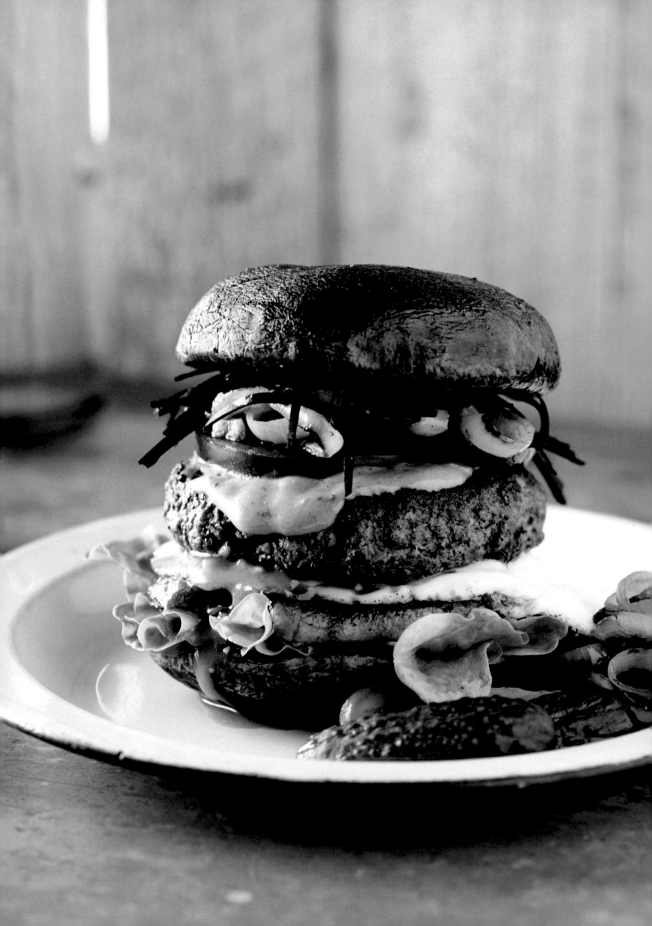

I can vividly remember arriving home from a long surf and feeling stoked to find my mum making burgers! To be honest, not a lot has changed since then. I still love going for long surfs and coming home to enjoy a juicy homemade burger. This recipe is basically the same as Mum used to make, but with portobello mushrooms instead of buns. The mushrooms might be a stretch for the kids, so omit the mushroom if the kids are fussy and just let them know that you're having a bun-free burger, which is just as yummy and way better for them. You can also try the Seed & Nut Bread (page 17) if you feel you still need bread. To jazz up the burgers, I've added homemade mayo, and fermented condiments and pickles.

MUM'S BURGERS

SERVES 4

8 large portobello mushrooms (remove the tough stems)

6 tbsp (80 g) coconut oil, melted, or duck, beef, or pork fat or ghee

1⅓ lb (600 g) minced beef chuck

½ brown onion, finely diced, plus 1 brown onion, sliced into rings

5 eggs

1 tbsp fermented mustard (page 206)

2 cloves garlic, finely chopped

1 tbsp chopped fresh flat-leaf parsley leaves

Pinch each of red chilli flakes and dried oregano

4 rashers nitrate-free bacon (optional)

condiments
8 butter lettuce leaves

8 ripe tomato slices

1 carrot, peeled and grated

1 beetroot, peeled and cut into thin matchsticks

4 pickles or gherkins, sliced

4 tbsp chipotle aïoli (page 203)

2 tbsp fermented ketchup (page 206) or homemade ketchup

2 tbsp fermented mustard (page 206) or other mustard you love

Preheat the oven to 450°F (240°C gas 8). Line a baking sheet with baking parchment, add the mushrooms gill side down, and drizzle with 3 tbsp coconut oil. Season with sea salt and freshly cracked black pepper, and bake for 10 to 15 minutes, until tender. Place the mushrooms on paper towels to remove the excess moisture, and let cool.

To make the patties, in a large bowl, mix together the beef, diced onion, 1 egg, mustard, garlic, parsley, red chilli flakes, oregano, 1 tsp sea salt, and 1 tsp freshly cracked black pepper. Shape into four patties about 3 inches (8 cm) in diameter and ½ inch (1.5 cm) thick.

Preheat a barbecue flatplate or heavy-based frying pan to medium heat. Add 2 tbsp coconut oil. Put the onion rings on the flatplate or pan and cook for about 10 minutes, stirring occasionally. Add the patties and bacon (if using), alongside the onions. Cook for 5 minutes or until golden, then flip the patties and bacon and continue cooking for a couple of minutes, until the meats are cooked through. The onion should be tender and caramelized. Remove the patties, bacon, and caramelized onions and set aside to keep warm.

In separate serving bowls, set out the lettuce, sliced tomatoes, grated carrot, beetroot, pickles, aïoli, ketchup, and mustard.

Add the remaining 1 tbsp oil to the barbecue flatplate or frying pan and fry the remaining 4 eggs to your liking. Season with salt and pepper.

Place the burgers, mushrooms, caramelized onions, and fried eggs in the middle of the table with the condiments and let each diner build his or her own burger.

This Middle Eastern-inspired recipe is ideal for many reasons. It is, of course, delicious and nutritious – and it's a favourite for my daughters. They love rolling the meatballs, and their nimble little hands have become much quicker than mine. We always make a huge batch so that we can pop them into school lunches and also enjoy them as leftovers or snacks for the next couple of days. The pomegranates and roast pumpkin really jazz this dish up into something special. It is divine to enjoy hot or cold.

LAMB MEATBALLS
WITH ROASTED PUMPKIN, POMEGRANATE & TAHINI SAUCE
SERVES 4

roasted pumpkin
½ pumpkin, fibre and seeds removed, flesh cut into 1-inch (2.5 cm) wedges

2 tbsp coconut oil, melted

2 pinches ground cumin

meatballs
14 oz (400 g) lean minced lamb

1 clove garlic, finely chopped

1 tomato, seeded and finely diced

1½ tbsp Turkish spice mix (page 206)

1 tbsp pomegranate molasses, plus more to serve

2 tbsp coconut oil

tahini sauce
½ cup (120 g) unhulled tahini paste

1 tbsp freshly squeezed lemon juice

1 tsp ground sumac

½ tsp ground cumin

1 small handful of fresh mint leaves, chopped

to serve
Extra virgin olive oil

2 pinches ground sumac

Roasted pumpkin seeds, activated (page 209)

Seeds of 1 pomegranate

2 handfuls of fresh mint leaves, torn

Lemon wedges

Preheat the oven to 400°F (200°C gas 6). On a baking sheet, drizzle the pumpkin wedges with the coconut oil and toss to coat evenly. Arrange the pumpkin in a single layer lying flat and sprinkle with sea salt, freshly cracked black pepper, and cumin. Roast for 20 to 25 minutes, until tender.

Meanwhile, combine the lamb with the garlic, tomato, Turkish spice mix, and pomegranate molasses in a bowl. Mix thoroughly and season with salt and pepper. Coat a baking sheet with 1 tbsp coconut oil. Shape the lamb mixture into walnut-size meatballs. In a large frying pan over medium heat, heat the remaining 1 tbsp coconut oil. Pan-fry the meatballs for 2 to 3 minutes, until browned. Place on the baking sheet in a single layer and bake until cooked through, about 5 minutes.

To make the sauce, combine the tahini, 4 tbsp water, lemon juice, sumac, cumin, and mint. Stir until smooth.

To serve, place the pumpkin on a serving platter, drizzle with a little olive oil and sprinkle with salt, pepper, sumac, pumpkin seeds, pomegranates seeds, and mint. Drizzle with some of the tahini sauce. Transfer the meatballs to a serving bowl, and drizzle with some pomegranate molasses. Serve with the remaining tahini sauce and lemon wedges alongside.

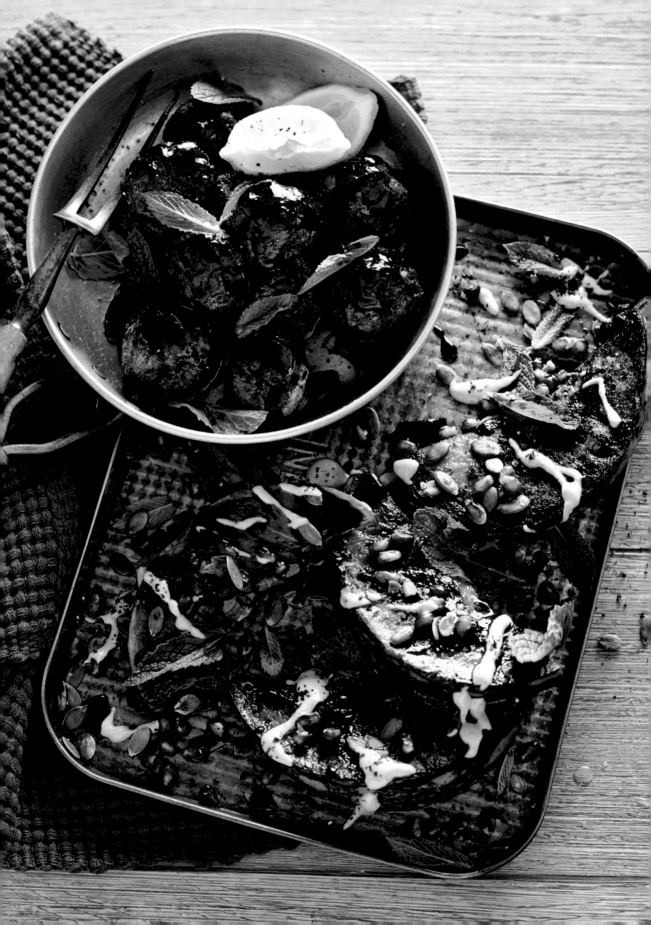

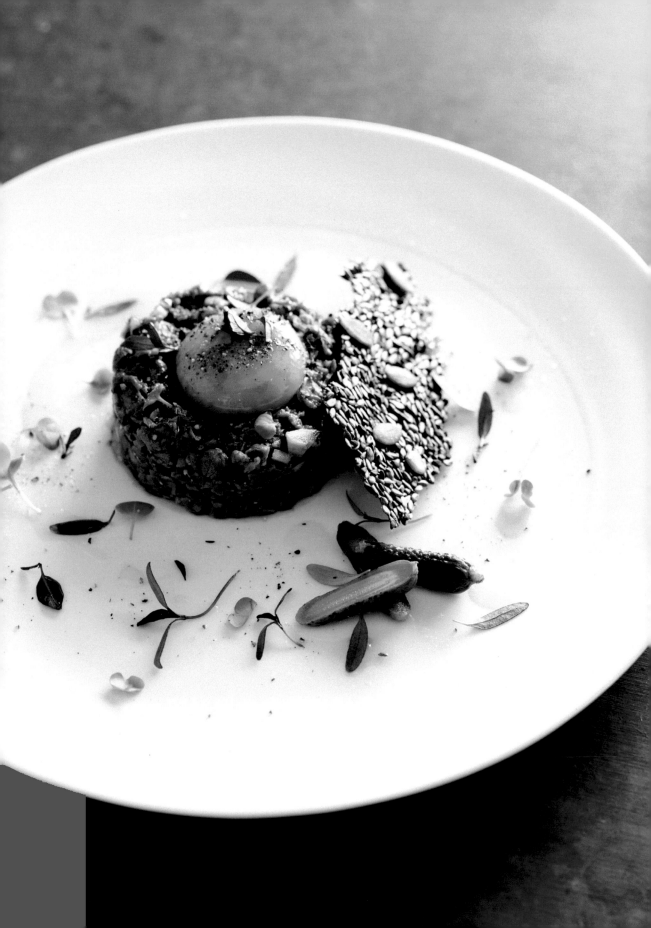

When dealing with raw meat, you have to be super clean and move quickly. To keep it chilled, it's a good idea to mix your ingredients in a cold stainless steel bowl over a bowl of ice; you can even put a couple of ice cubes into the mix to keep it cold. My partner, Nic, and I usually eat a raw protein dish twice a week for dinner in the warmer months, and we can have it on the table in less than 15 minutes. We always change our ingredients; sometimes it's mayonnaise-based and sometimes we just use olive oil and lemon juice or vinegar to dress the meat. We also flavour it with horseradish, wasabi, harissa, *chermoula*, jerk seasoning, or coconut cream. We love this particular dish because it takes no time at all and the flavour combinations are endless.

STEAK TARTARE
SERVES 4

1 tbsp fermented mustard (page 206)

4 salt-packed anchovy fillets, rinsed well and patted dry then finely chopped

2 tbsp fermented ketchup (page 206)

Tabasco sauce

3 tbsp extra virgin olive oil

¼ cup (45 g) capers, rinsed

4 tbsp finely chopped red onion

8 cornichons, finely chopped, plus more to serve

1 small handful of fresh flat-leaf parsley leaves, finely chopped

Juice of 1 lemon

14 oz (400 g) fillet steak, very finely chopped

4 egg yolks

Fresh micro herbs, to garnish

Seed crackers (page 207), to serve

Mix the mustard and anchovies in a large stainless steel bowl. Add the ketchup, and some Tabasco, and freshly cracked black pepper and mix well. Slowly whisk in the oil. Fold in the capers, onion, cornichons, parsley, lemon juice and a little sea salt. Add the meat to the bowl and mix well with a spoon or your hands.

Serve on four plates, using a 2½-inch (7 cm) ring mould to shape the meat into neat circles. Make a small hollow on the top of each one with a spoon and place an egg yolk in it. Sprinkle with the micro herbs and season with salt and pepper. Serve with the crackers and cornichons.

I don't eat a lot of pork. It isn't that I don't like it; in fact, it's quite the opposite. I love it. I have a bit of a weakness for it, so I am diligent in the amount that I consume, otherwise it would be on my plate daily. My favourite ways to cook pork are to either roast a shoulder with rosemary and sea salt, braise some pork belly in an Asian-inspired broth, make a terrine using the whole head, or stuff the trotters (a bit time-consuming, but well worth the effort). Of course, I can't forget about pork and fennel sausages, or blood pudding, or amazing chorizo. Okay, you get the picture: pork tastes great, and this recipe is a terrific way to eat it! Remember to always hunt down free-range pork that has had a natural diet.

PORK CUTLETS
WITH CABBAGE SALAD & ROMESCO SAUCE
SERVES 4

cabbage salad
½ cup (125 ml) extra virgin olive oil

3½ tbsp (100 ml) Chardonnay vinegar

¼ head Savoy cabbage

2¼ cups (200 g) brussels sprouts

1 cup (150 g) almonds, activated (page 209), toasted, and chopped

1 handful of fresh flat-leaf parsley leaves, finely chopped

1 handful of fresh mint leaves, finely chopped

4 bone-in pork chops, each about 10 oz (300 g) and ¾ inch (2 cm) thick

2 tbsp coconut oil, ghee, or duck fat, melted

½ cup (120 ml) romesco sauce (page 204)

To make the salad, whisk the olive oil and vinegar in a bowl and set aside. Discard the outer leaves of the cabbage. Shave the cabbage and the brussels sprouts finely with a sharp knife or a mandoline, discarding any thick ribs from the cabbage. Combine the cabbage and brussels sprouts in a large bowl with the toasted almonds, parsley, and mint. Add half of the vinaigrette, season with sea salt and freshly cracked black pepper, then toss together gently. Allow the salad to stand for up to 10 minutes.

Meanwhile, coat the pork chops with the coconut oil and season with salt and pepper. Heat a frying pan over medium-high heat and cook the pork chops on each side until cooked through, 4 minutes per side. Remove from the heat and allow to rest for 2 minutes.

Spread the romesco sauce on four serving plates, dividing it evenly. Top each with a pork chop and some of the salad, and serve.

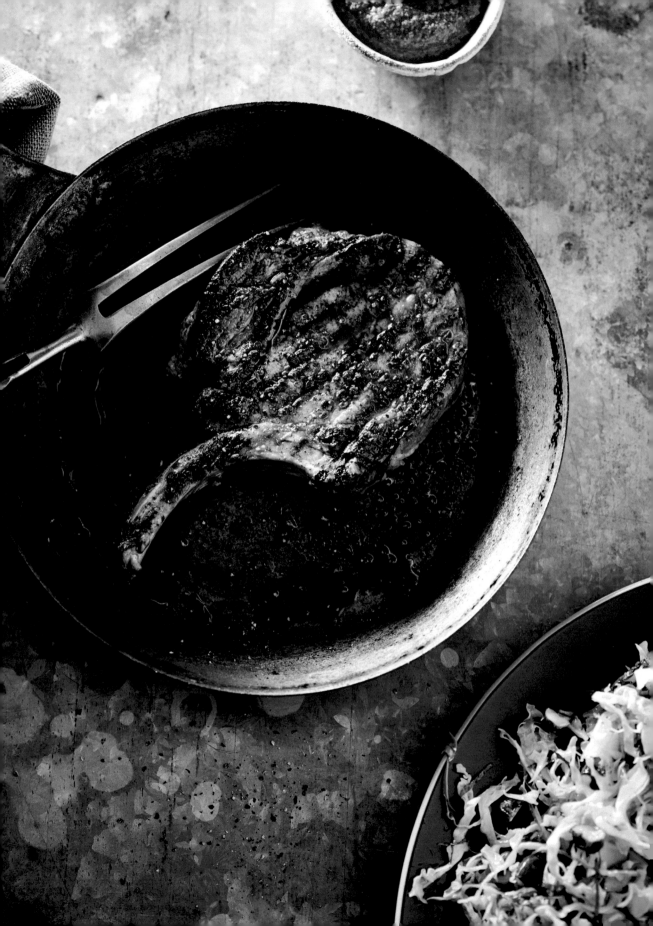

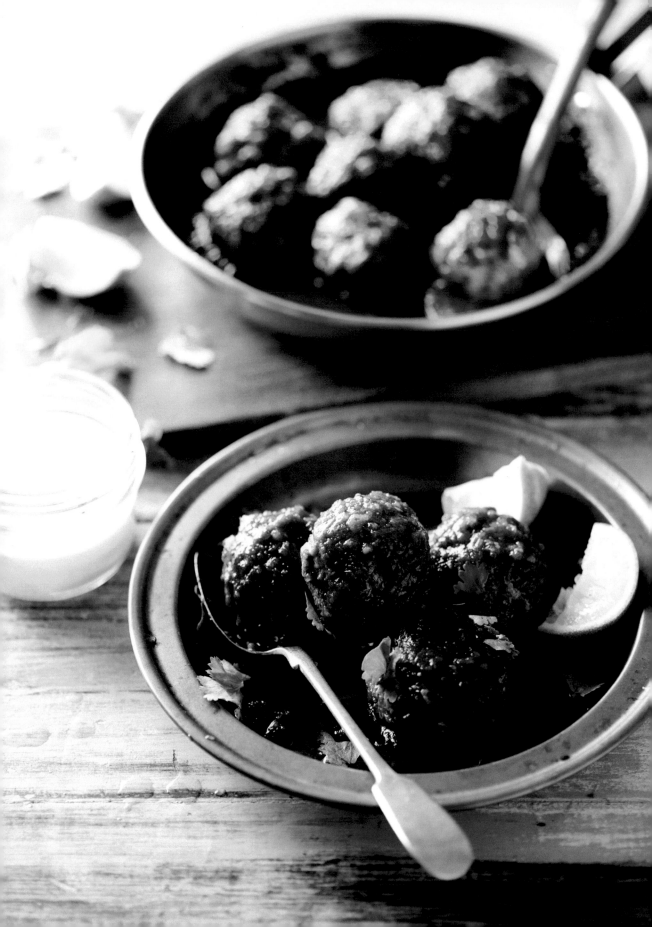

These meatballs are a hit in our household and are often requested by my children because they are so full of flavour. They love eating them, and they like helping to make them, too. We make extra so that the kids can take them to school the next day. This recipe uses chipotles in adobo sauce, so be sure to look for a brand that is organic and sugar-free. I have also included a dairy-free version of Mexican *crema*, which is usually made with cream, but I have used cashews (which you can replace with macadamia nuts, if desired). It should go without saying that if you are feeding this to the kids, don't make it too spicy for them.

MEATBALLS IN CHIPOTLE SAUCE
SERVES 4

meatballs
12 oz (350 g) minced pork

12 oz (350 g) minced beef

1 egg

2 tbsp dried oregano

2 tsp ground cumin

4 cloves garlic, finely chopped

1 tbsp chopped fresh
flat-leaf parsley

2 tbsp coconut oil, ghee,
or duck fat

chipotle sauce
1 cup (7 oz/200 g) canned
whole peeled tomatoes

1 onion, chopped

2 (7 oz/198 g) cans chipotle
chillies in adobo sauce

1 tsp tomato paste

2 tbsp raw honey (optional)

1 tbsp extra virgin olive oil

1 cup (250 ml) chicken stock
(page 202)

dairy-free mexican *crema*
1½ cups (210 g) raw cashews
or macadamia nuts

Juice of 1 lemon

Juice of 1 lime

Fresh coriander leaves, to garnish

Lime wedges, to serve

To make the meatballs, combine the pork and beef in a large bowl. Add the egg, oregano, cumin, garlic, parsley, 2 tsp sea salt, and ¼ tsp freshly cracked black pepper. Mix well with your hands until the ingredients are well blended. To form the meatballs, place 1 tbsp of the meat mixture in the palm of your hand and, moving both hands together in a circular motion, form a 1½-inch (3 cm) ball. Set aside and repeat until you have used all the meat.

In a large saucepan, heat the coconut oil over a medium-high heat. Add the meatballs in batches and sear the meatballs until golden brown, 1 to 2 minutes. Transfer to a plate and set aside; the meatballs don't need be cooked through at this stage.

To make the chipotle sauce, combine the tomatoes, onion, chipotles, 1 tbsp of the adobo sauce, tomato paste, honey, if using, and olive oil in a blender and puree. Pour the mixture into the same saucepan that you used for the meatballs and bring to the boil. Reduce the heat and simmer for 10 minutes. Pour in the stock and bring back to the boil. Add the meatballs and cook for 10 minutes. They can stay in the sauce until you are ready to serve.

To make the *crema*, combine the cashews, ¾ cup (200 ml) water, lemon juice, and lime juice in a food processor and process until smooth. Season to taste with salt.

Transfer the meatballs and sauce to a serving bowl and sprinkle with coriander. Serve with the chipotle sauce, *crema*, and lime wedges.

There isn't a lot to this recipe: it is basically a tomato and herb salad that is served alongside excellent grass-fed beef. But it can be on the table in minutes for lunch or dinner and is utterly delicious from the first mouthful to the last. Serve it with a big bowl of green vegetables to make it a complete meal, or chop up some avocado and toss it into the tomato salad to add some beneficial fat to keep you satiated longer.

GRILLED SIRLOIN
WITH TOMATO-HERB SALAD

SERVES 4

salad
½ cup (125 ml) extra virgin olive oil

⅓ cup (80 ml) raw apple cider vinegar or sherry vinegar

1½ lb (700 g) mixed vine-ripened heirloom tomatoes, cut into thin wedges

1 cup (120 g) marinated olives (page 208)

2 tbsp capers, rinsed

1 bunch of chives, chopped

Leaves from 1 bunch of basil

4 (5½ oz/150 g) sirloin or beef tenderloin steaks

2 tbsp coconut oil, melted

to serve
A few handfuls of rocket

Extra virgin olive oil

Lemon wedges

1 tsp fried garlic, crushed (page 207)

To make the salad, in a large bowl, whisk together the olive oil and vinegar. Add the tomatoes, olives, capers, and chives to the bowl. Season with sea salt and freshly cracked black pepper, toss gently to combine, and allow it to marinate for 5 to 10 minutes. Add the basil and toss together.

Rub the steaks with coconut oil and season with salt and pepper. Preheat a barbecue or grill pan to high heat. Add the steaks and cook for 2 minutes on each side, or until cooked to your liking. Let rest for 3 minutes.

To serve, in a bowl, toss together the rocket, a drizzle of olive oil, and a squeeze of lemon. Place a steak on each of four plates, arrange the tomato salad on top, and sprinkle with the crushed fried garlic and a few grinds of pepper. Serve with the dressed rocket and lemon wedges alongside.

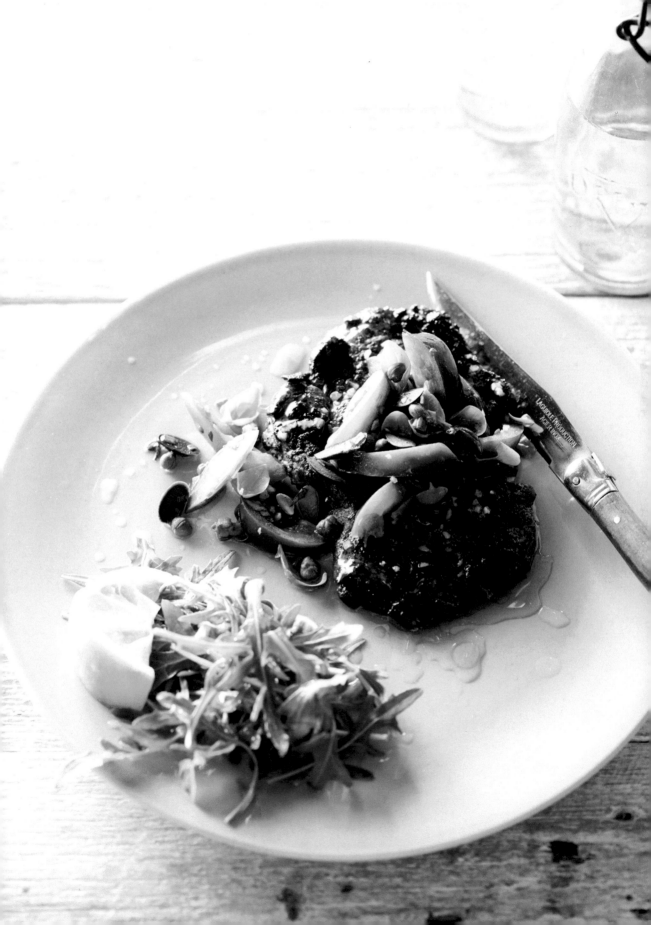

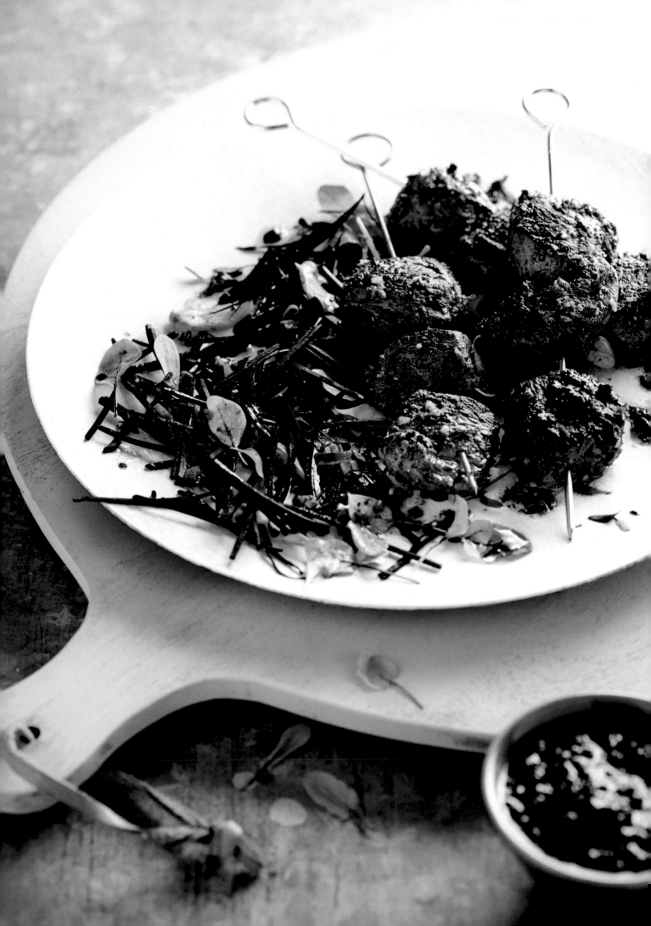

Venison has a delicious gamey flavour that is stronger than beef but equally as wonderful. I love cooking with it. Just as with lean cuts of beef, it is important to not overcook it, or the lean meat will be dry. I often enjoy my venison rare unless I am making a braise from the secondary cuts. You can use heart, liver, steak, or even minced meat for these skewers. The chimichurri sauce works well with pretty much any protein; I have added some beetroot to it because beetroot and game work hand in hand, and give the plate lovely colour.

VENISON SKEWERS
WITH BEETROOT CHIMICHURRI
SERVES 4

beetroot chimichurri

1 large beetroot, peeled and grated

1 cup (250 ml) extra virgin olive oil, plus more as needed

1 cup (60 g) loosely packed fresh flat-leaf parsley leaves

½ red onion, chopped

2 cloves garlic, finely chopped

4 tbsp chopped fresh oregano

4 tbsp raw apple cider vinegar or red wine vinegar

½ tsp red chilli flakes

venison

1¾ lb (800 g) venison, cut into 1-inch (3 cm) cubes

½ cup (100 g) ghee, lard, or coconut oil, melted

1 tbsp finely grated lemon zest

3 tbsp freshly squeezed lemon juice

4 tbsp chopped fresh oregano

2 cloves garlic, finely chopped

1½ tsp ground cumin

½ tsp ground fennel

½ tsp ground coriander

salad

4 tbsp extra virgin olive oil

1 tbsp balsamic vinegar

1 large beetroot, peeled and cut into thin matchsticks

1 handful of baby red-veined sorrel or beetroot leaves

Grated fresh horseradish, to serve

Soak eight bamboo skewers in water for 30 minutes. To make the chimichurri sauce, combine the grated beetroot, oil, parsley, onion, garlic, oregano, vinegar, and red chilli flakes in a food processer and pulse until finely chopped. Add a little more oil if the sauce is too thick. Season with sea salt and freshly cracked black pepper.

Thread five to six pieces of venison on each skewer, place in a deep dish, and set aside.

Combine the ghee, lemon zest, 2 tbsp lemon juice, oregano, garlic, cumin, fennel, and coriander in a bowl and whisk together. Pour over the venison and turn to evenly coat. Cover with plastic wrap and refrigerate for 1 hour to develop the flavours.

Preheat a grill pan or barbecue to high. Arrange the skewers on the grill pan or barbecue and cook for 2 to 3 minutes on each side, making sure the meat is slightly pink in the centre (or cook it to your liking). Season with salt and pepper and finish with the remaining 1 tbsp lemon juice. Remove from the heat and allow to rest for 2 minutes, keeping it warm, before serving.

Meanwhile, to make the salad, whisk together the oil and vinegar in a bowl. Add the beetroot and sorrel, toss gently, and season with salt and pepper.

To serve, place the venison skewers on a platter and grate horseradish over the top. Serve with the chimichurri and salad.

Michelle Tam, the founder of the wonderful website nomnompaleo.com, is truly a generous and gracious human being who knows how to make cooking fun, informative, and not scary for everyday cooks who want to implement a Paleo approach to their lives. Michelle includes her gorgeous family in her posts and in her book, *Nom Nom Paleo*, as well as step-by-step pictures of the dishes she makes. She also provides a wealth of knowledge in the tips. Michelle has kindly shared one of my favourite dishes of hers: these surf and turf tacos. Keep cooking with love and laughter — I am sure Michelle and her family always will.

NOM NOM PALEO'S SURF & TURF TACOS

SERVES 4

guacamole
1 large avocado

Juice of 1 lime

1 to 2 tbsp finely diced red onion

1 tbsp chopped fresh coriander leaves

2 tbsp extra virgin olive oil

2 to 3 pinches Aleppo pepper (optional)

2 tbsp ghee, coconut oil, or macadamia nut oil

1 lb (500 g) minced beef

2 pinches of Penzeys Spices chilli 9000 or your favourite chilli powder

12 medium prawns, peeled and de-veined, tails left on

2 pinches of *tabil* (Tunisian spice blend; page 206)

1 head baby romaine lettuce, leaves separated

1 carrot, peeled and julienned

12 cherry tomatoes, halved

¼ bunch of coriander, chopped

To make the guacamole, halve the avocado, discard the stone, and scoop out the avocado flesh into a bowl. Mash with a fork. Stir in the lime juice, onion, coriander, and olive oil. Season with sea salt and freshly cracked black pepper. Sprinkle with Aleppo pepper, if using. Set aside.

Heat a frying pan with 1 tbsp of the ghee over medium heat. Add the beef and sauté until the meat is brown and cooked through, 8 to 10 minutes. Add the chilli powder and season with salt and pepper. Set aside.

In another frying pan over medium heat, heat the remaining 1 tbsp ghee. Cook the prawns for 1 minute on each side, until cooked through. Season with the *tabil*, salt, and pepper.

To serve, put the lettuce leaves on a serving platter or four plates, then top with meat, guacamole, and prawns. Finish with carrots, cherry tomatoes, and coriander.

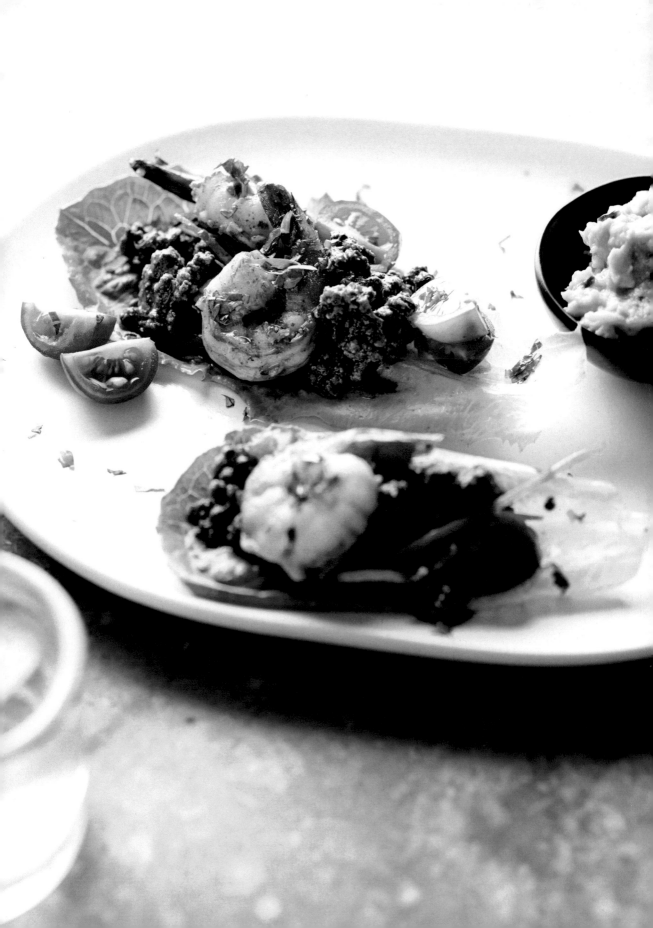

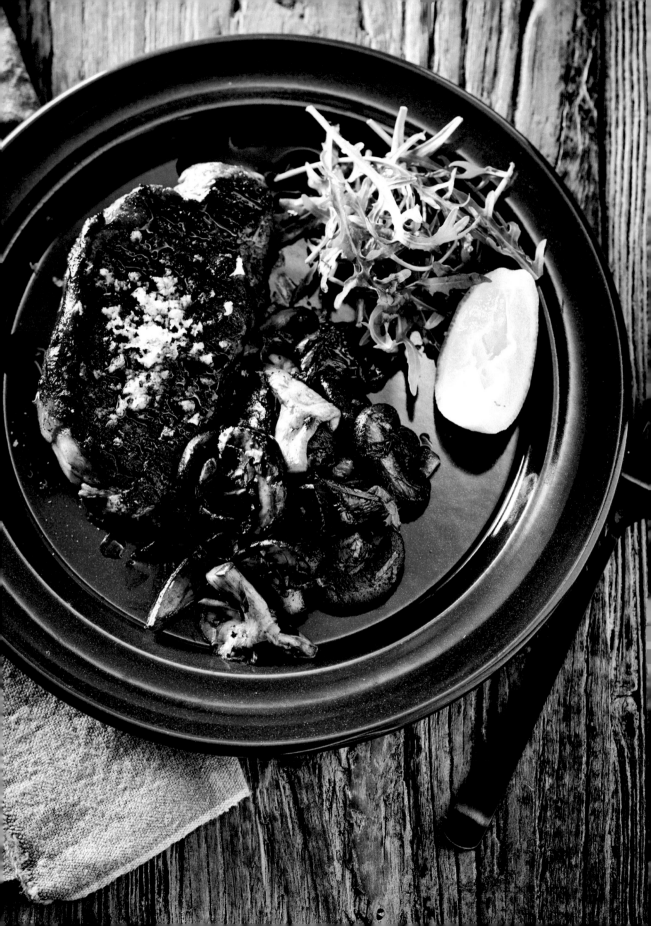

I am not a huge fan of steak and prefer raw meat (such as Steak Tartare on page 143); long, slow braises and curries using secondary cuts; or, even better, organ meats (which I find taste more exciting). A classic steak is cut from the leanest parts of the animal, and I find the meat to be the least flavourful and the hardest to chew and swallow. However, for anyone discovering the Paleo way of eating, it's a good idea to start with familiar dishes such as this: a sirloin or porterhouse or other prime cut that is well seasoned and cooked to your liking (mine is very rare), then topped with freshly grated horseradish, sautéed mushrooms, and a simple rocket salad. If I'm going to eat steak, this is how I like to prepare it.

GRILLED SIRLOIN
WITH MUSHROOMS, HORSERADISH & ROCKET
SERVES 4

4 (7 oz/200 g) sirloin steaks

2 tbsp ghee, coconut oil, or duck fat, melted

5 oz (150 g) chestnut mushrooms, sliced

3½ oz (100 g) oyster mushrooms, sliced

2 cloves garlic, finely chopped

3 sprigs thyme, chopped

1 tbsp chopped fresh flat-leaf parsley

1 tbsp freshly grated horseradish

2 handfuls of wild rocket

3 tbsp extra virgin olive oil or macadamia nut oil

2 lemons, cut into wedges

Preheat a grill pan or barbecue to high heat. Coat the meat with a little ghee and season with sea salt and freshly cracked black pepper. Put the meat in the grill pan or on the barbecue, and cook on one side for 4 minutes, or until browned, then flip the meat over and cook for another 4 minutes, until browned and medium-rare. Remove from the heat, place the meat on a tray or plate, and cover with aluminium foil. Allow the steaks to rest for 4 to 6 minutes and keep warm.

Meanwhile, in a frying pan over high heat, heat the remaining ghee. Add the mushrooms, garlic, and thyme and sauté until the mushrooms are cooked through, 2 to 4 minutes. Season with salt and pepper. Stir in the parsley, remove from the heat, and cover to keep warm.

Once the steaks are well rested, reheat the steaks by placing them back in the grill pan or on the barbecue for 1 minute on both sides. Place on four serving plates, then sprinkle the steaks with the freshly grated horseradish.

Toss the rocket with the olive oil and a squeeze of lemon juice and season with salt and pepper. Place on top of the steaks and serve with the sautéed mushrooms and lemon wedges.

Piri piri (also *peri peri*) sauce is a spicy, fragrant Portuguese favourite that is often served on roasted butterflied chicken. It is nothing short of spectacular. I am always looking for ways to turn cheaper cuts of meat, especially minced meat, into flavourful sensations, and I often incorporate sauces and marinades that I have tasted on my travels, like *piri piri*. Purchase minced pork from a respected butcher who will mince it for you or order it online from a purveyor that only has free-range pigs on a natural diet. It is important to source ethically raised pigs that weren't fed GMO soy protein or other nasties. Make extra *piri piri* sauce because, like me, once you try it, you will no doubt start putting it on everything.

PORTUGUESE PORK BURGERS
WITH PIRI PIRI SAUCE
SERVES 6

piri piri sauce
1 tbsp coconut oil

2 tbsp sweet paprika

1 tbsp ground cumin

1 tbsp ground coriander

1 red pepper, seeded and chopped

½ brown onion, chopped

2 fresh red chillies, seeded

1 tsp peeled and grated ginger

Juice of 1 lemon

⅔ cup (150 ml) extra virgin olive oil

burgers
1¾ lb (800 g) coarsely minced pork shoulder

1 egg

3 cloves garlic, finely chopped

1 tsp chilli powder, such as ancho

1 tsp dried oregano

1 lemon, halved

Baby romaine lettuce, leaves separated

½ cup (120 ml) aïoli (page 203)

Hot paprika, for garnish (optional)

To make the *piri piri* sauce, combine the coconut oil, paprika, cumin, and coriander in a frying pan over medium heat and cook until fragrant, 1 minute. Add the red pepper, onion, chillies, and ginger and cook until soft and translucent, 3 minutes. Mix in the lemon juice. Transfer the mixture to a blender and blend until smooth. Pour in the olive oil in a slow, steady stream while blending until the oil is incorporated in the sauce. Season with sea salt and freshly cracked black pepper.

To make the burgers, combine the pork, egg, garlic, chilli powder, oregano, 1 tbsp salt, and 1½ tsp black pepper in a mixing bowl and knead for 1 minute until well combined. Form the pork mixture into 12 golf ball–size rounds, then gently press into patties that are about 1 inch (2.5 cm) thick.

Preheat a grill pan or barbecue to medium heat. Add the patties and cook for 3 to 4 minutes on each side, or until cooked through. Grill the lemon halves for 1 minute, or until caramelized.

To serve, place the burgers on lettuce cups, spoon over some *piri piri* and aïoli, and finish with a squeeze of caramelized lemon and a sprinkle of paprika.

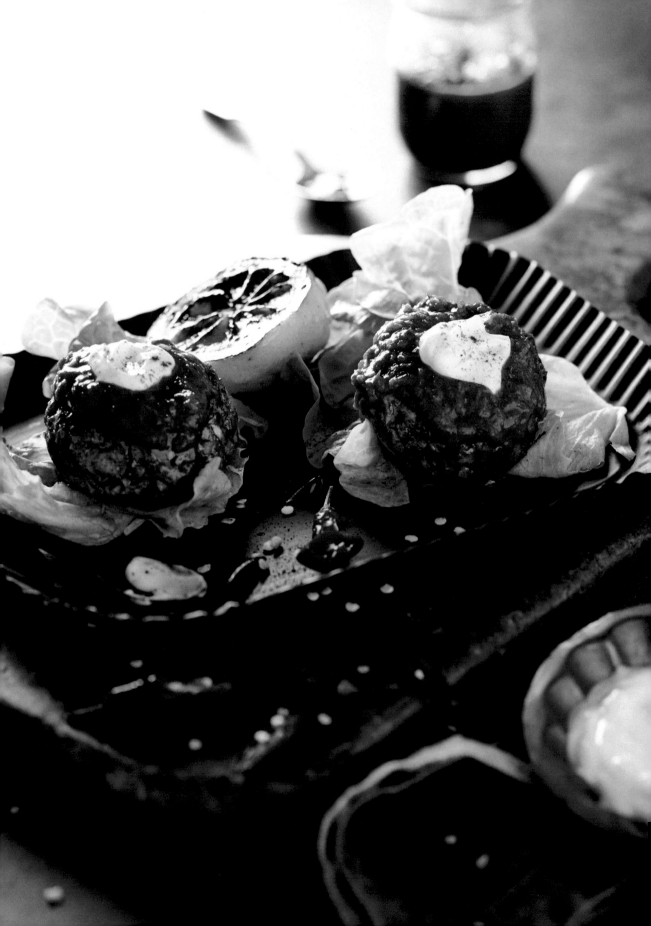

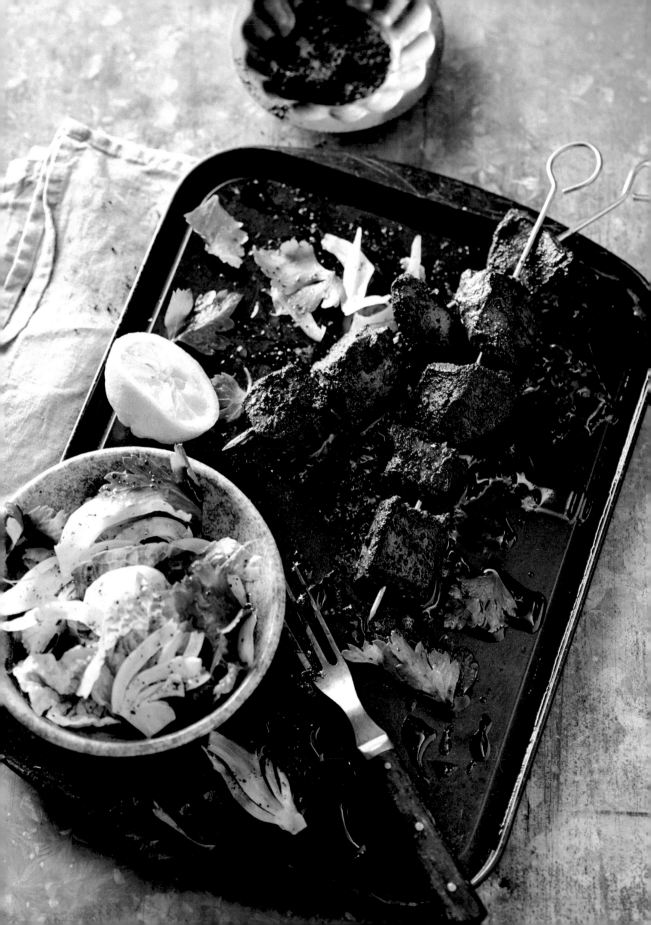

Many of us are aware that we should be eating nose-to-tail, and my challenge is to make those bits taste even better than the prime cuts we are used to eating. If that can happen, then not only will you be saving a fortune at the butcher, but your body will be thanking you for giving it the nutrients it needs. I wanted to add some excitement to these kebabs by using some serious spices to marinate or coat them in, so I chose harissa, one of my favourite sauces. Harissa, which hails from North Africa, is a blend of spices that have been cooked down with chillies and peppers to form a pungent yet thoroughly addictive paste that enhances any type of meat or vegetable.

LAMB LIVER KEBABS
WITH SUMAC & PARSLEY SALAD

SERVES 4

1¾ lb (800 g) lambs' liver or calves' liver

2 tbsp harissa (page 205)

1½ tbsp ground sumac

1½ tbsp ground cumin

½ tsp sweet paprika

6 tbsp (80 g) ghee or coconut oil, melted

salad
1 head baby romaine lettuce, torn

1 fennel bulb, shaved

½ cup (30 g) fresh flat-leaf parsley leaves

dressing
Freshly squeezed juice from ½ lemon

3 tbsp extra virgin olive oil

1 tsp ground sumac

Lemon, to serve

Use your fingers to remove the membrane from the livers, then cut out any little tubes with a small sharp knife. Cut the trimmed liver into ¾-inch (2 cm) cubes.

Combine the harissa, sumac, cumin, paprika, and ghee in a bowl. Add the liver and toss gently to coat. Set aside for 30 minutes to marinate.

Meanwhile, if using bamboo skewers, soak eight skewers in water for 30 minutes prior to using.

To make the salad, in a large bowl, toss together the lettuce, fennel, and parsley and set aside. To make the dressing, combine the lemon juice, olive oil, sumac, and a pinch of sea salt, and mix well until combined. Set aside.

When you are ready to cook, preheat a grill pan or barbecue to high heat. Thread four cubes of liver onto eight skewers. Cook for 20 to 30 seconds on each side; season with salt and freshly cracked black pepper.

Remove the skewers from the grill. Toss the salad with the sumac dressing and arrange the salad on four serving plates. Top the salad with two skewers on each and squeeze over a good amount of lemon juice to finish.

Liver is one of my favourite parts of the cow. It is one of the most nutritionally dense and most often overlooked or misunderstood ingredients. People often expect liver to be heavy and unappealing. Bearing that in mind, I have tried to keep this recipe light and fresh by using a lively vinaigrette as my sauce. The vinaigrette includes a generous amount of vinegar, which brings some much-needed acidity to the rich meat. It also makes it possible to bring in fresh ingredients that complement the liver, like greens and fresh figs.

SEARED BEEF LIVER
WITH FIG SALAD & SHERRY VINAIGRETTE
SERVES 4

sherry vinaigrette
1 small red onion, chopped

Ghee or coconut oil, for cooking

3 tbsp raw apple cider vinegar or sherry vinegar

1 tbsp fermented mustard (page 206)

3 tbsp cold-pressed walnut oil (optional)

7 tbsp (100 ml) extra virgin olive oil

fig salad
7 oz (200 g) pancetta, thinly sliced

1 head frisée

1 cup (100 g) walnuts, activated (page 209), toasted and chopped

6 fresh figs, cut into wedges

liver
4 (5½ oz/150 g) slices beef liver

2 tbsp coconut oil or beef or duck fat

To make the sherry vinaigrette, in a small saucepan over low heat, gently cook the onion with a little ghee until soft, about 5 minutes. Add the vinegar and set aside to cool. Transfer to a bowl and whisk in the mustard, then the walnut oil, if using, and olive oil. Set aside.

To make the salad, in a large frying pan over medium-high heat, cook the pancetta until crisp, about 3 minutes, turning once. Drain on paper towels, then crumble.

Prepare the frisée by cutting out the core and removing the darker outer leaves; use only use the lighter centre leaves for this dish. In a large bowl, toss together the frisée, pancetta, and walnuts. Set aside.

Season the liver with sea salt and freshly cracked black pepper. In the frying pan over medium-high heat, warm the coconut oil. When the oil is hot, add the liver and cook, turning once, until still slightly pink in the middle or cooked to your liking, 4 to 6 minutes.

Drizzle the salad with some of the vinaigrette, add the figs, and gently toss together. Serve the liver topped with the salad, passing any remaining vinaigrette alongside.

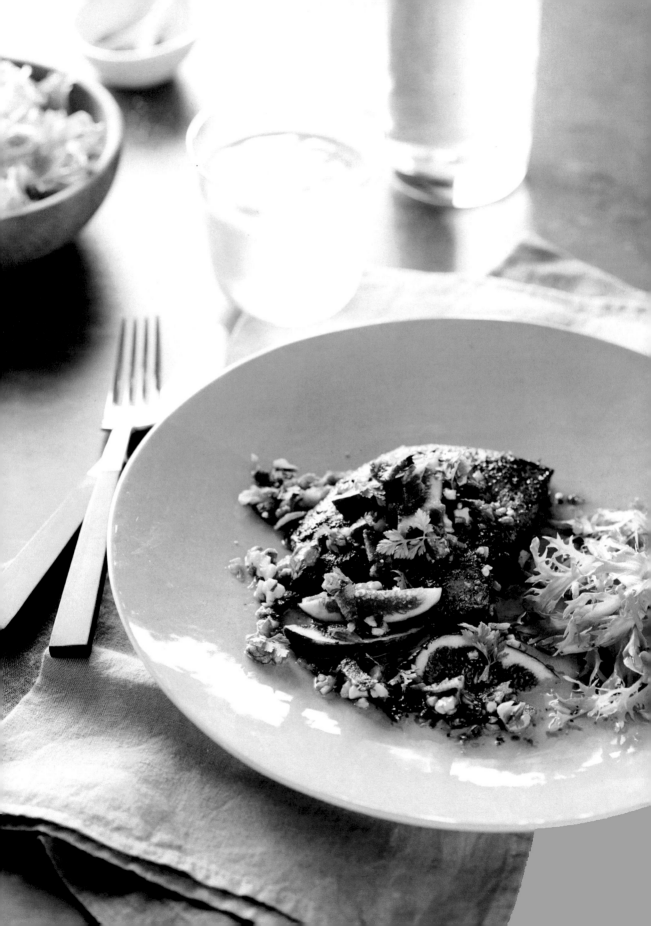

DESSERT

Key lime tart is a favourite, so I came up with a gorgeous Paleo version. Fortunately, I've got friends and family who are always up for a recipe-tasting session when I'm creating new desserts, and I'm pleased to say that this dessert got two thumbs up all the way. I have yet to meet someone who hasn't got a soft spot for a delicious citrus tart, and none can be more delicious than this version. I hope you enjoy it!

KEY LIME TART

SERVES 8 TO 10

candied lime
2 limes, thinly sliced
¾ cup (255 g) raw honey

crust
1 cup (160 g) almonds, activated (page 209)

⅔ cup (90 g) unsweetened shredded dried coconut

6 medjool dates, pitted

1 vanilla bean, split lengthwise and scraped

2 tbsp coconut oil

filling
3 ripe avocados

¾ cup (175 ml) freshly squeezed lime juice

¾ cup (255 g) raw honey

½ cup (125 g) coconut oil

To make the candied lime, bring a saucepan of water to a boil, add the limes, and blanch for a few seconds. Drain and plunge into a bowl of ice water. Repeat this process twice more. Combine 1 cup (250 ml) water and the honey in a small saucepan over high heat. Bring to a boil, stirring to combine. Add the blanched limes, reduce the heat, and gently simmer until the limes become translucent, 40 to 60 minutes. Allow to cool completely in the syrup. Store in the syrup in a sterilized airtight jar in the refrigerator for up to 3 months.

Meanwhile, to make the crust, combine the almonds and coconut in a food processor and process until broken up into a nice crumble. Add the dates, vanilla bean seeds, coconut oil, and a pinch of sea salt, and pulse until the mixture just comes together. Press the dough firmly and evenly into a 4½ by 13¾-inch (12 by 35 cm) rectangular tart tin with a removable bottom (alternatively, you can use a 12-inch/30 cm round tart tin) to form the crust. Refrigerate for at least 1 hour, or until firm.

To make the filling, combine the avocados, lime juice, honey, coconut oil, and ⅛ tsp salt in a blender. Blend until smooth. Adjust the flavours to taste.

Pour the filling into the crust, spread it into a smooth, even layer, and chill for at least 4 hours, or overnight. Garnish with the candied lime slices and serve.

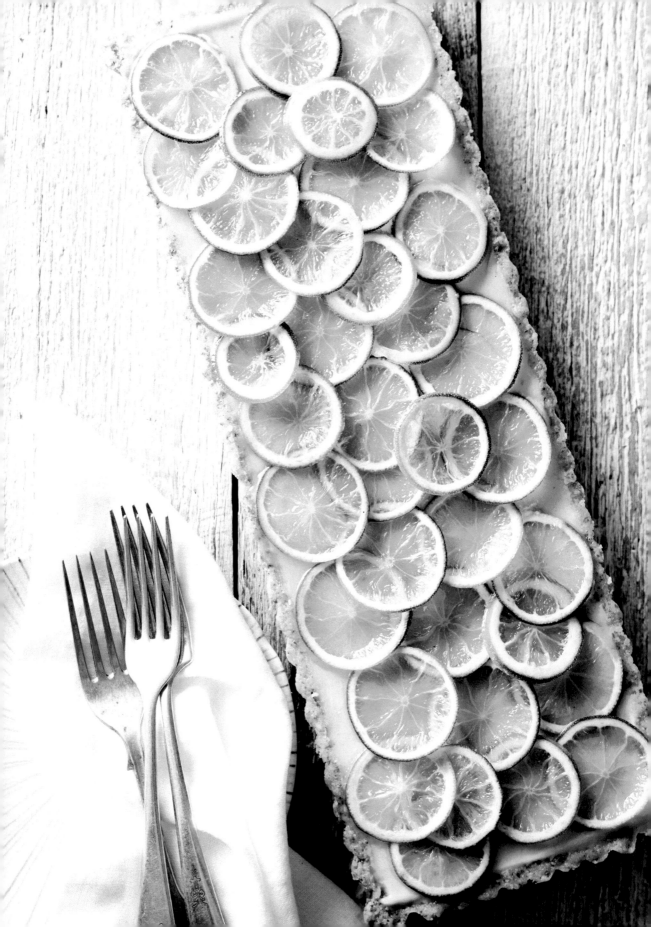

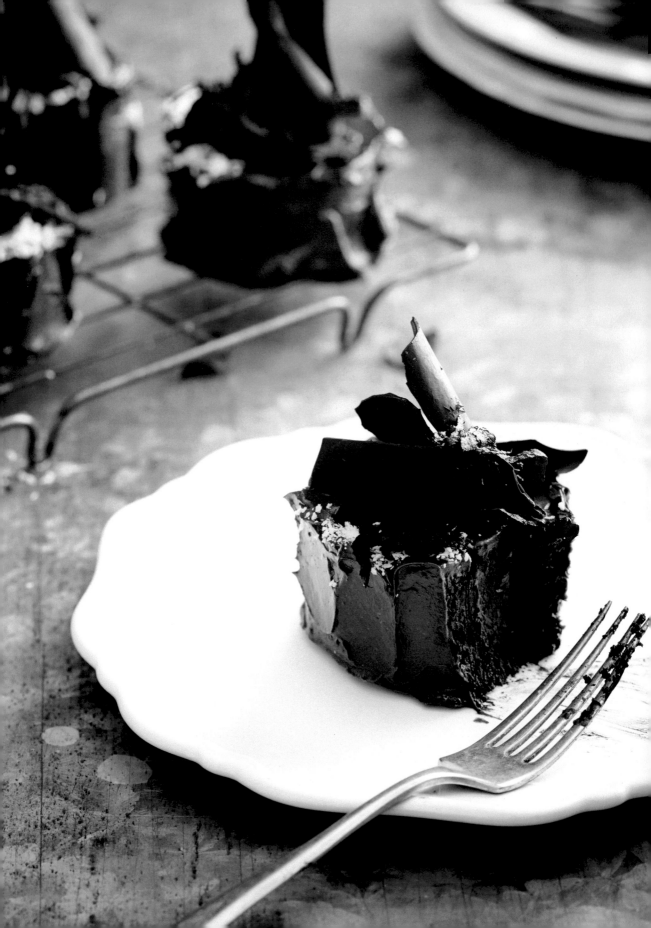

I love making raw foods, so experimenting with ingredients to make this cake worthy was a true labour of love. The initial inspiration for these little cakes came from Dr Libby Weaver, a holistic nutrition expert, and her delicious recipe for raw beetroot muffins. It was rather good, but adding chocolate to the mix was, in my mind, the way to make it extra delicious and, of course, somewhat decadent. The colour of the cakes is as mesmerizing as the flavour, and the fact that there's no cooking involved means that the beetroot retains all of its goodness and natural enzymes.

CHOCOLATE BEETROOT MUDCAKES
SERVES 8

mudcake
2 cups (300 g) mixed macadamia nuts and Brazil nuts, activated (page 209)

6 medjool dates

¼ cup (40 g) dried currants, dried blueberries, or dried cranberries

⅓ cup (70 ml) maple syrup

3 beetroots, peeled and grated, plus more to serve

2¼ cups (200 g) unsweetened shredded dried coconut, plus more to serve

4 tbsp raw cacao powder

4 tbsp carob powder

½ tsp vanilla powder or 1 vanilla bean, split lengthwise and scraped

2 tbsp golden linseed meal

icing
2 avocados, halved, pitted, and peeled

½ cup (60 g) raw cacao powder

½ cup (170 g) raw honey

2 tbsp coconut oil

½ tsp vanilla powder

chocolate shavings
½ cup (120 ml) coconut oil, melted

1½ tbsp raw cacao powder, sifted

1½ tbsp carob powder, sifted

1 tbsp raw honey

To make the mudcakes, in a food processor, process the nuts to the consistency of bread-crumbs. Add the dates, currants, and maple syrup and process until smooth. Add the grated beetroot, coconut, cacao powder, carob powder, vanilla powder, and linseed meal and blend until well combined and even in texture. Line a baking sheet with baking parchment. Place eight 2 by 2-inch (5 by 5 cm) cake ring moulds on the baking sheet. Divide the nut-beetroot mixture among the moulds and place in the freezer for about 40 minutes to firm up.

To make the icing, blend the avocados, cacao powder, honey, coconut oil, vanilla, and ½ tsp sea salt in a clean food processor and pulse until smooth. Using a palette knife, cover the cakes with the icing. Place the cakes in the fridge for 30 minutes.

To make the chocolate shavings, mix the coconut oil, cacao powder, carob powder, and honey in a bowl. Line a baking sheet with baking parchment and spread the mixture onto the paper as thinly as possible. Leave at room temperature for 5 minutes, then carefully roll the paper to form a cylinder and place in the refrigerator for at least 10 minutes and up to 20 minutes to harden. Once the chocolate has hardened, peel the paper away; you will be left with pretty chocolate shavings. Place these on the baking sheet and return them to the refrigerator for another 2 to 5 minutes to firm up again.

Garnish the mudcakes with dried coconut, grated beetroot, and chocolate shavings and serve.

Cheesecake is a dessert I've never been able to take pleasure in because I'm lactose-intolerant, so this dairy-free version is right up my alley. Cashew nuts are a surprising yet marvellous substitute for the cream cheese in the filling, and in my opinion they're much more appetizing, too. The berries add an appealing contrast to the creamy cashew cheese. You can use macadamia nuts instead of cashews — just add a few tablespoons of water to the puree to get them to the same smooth consistency as the cashews.

MIXED BERRY CHEESECAKE
SERVES 6 TO 8

crumble

1 cup (160 g) almonds, activated (page 209)

1 cup (90 g) unsweetened shredded dried coconut

1 vanilla bean, split lengthwise and scraped

6 medjool dates, pitted

cheesecake

1 lb (450 g) cashews, soaked 4 to 6 hours, then drained and rinsed

½ cup (125 ml) freshly squeezed lime juice

¾ cup plus 2 tbsp (300 g) raw honey

1 vanilla bean, split lengthwise and scraped

1 cup (250 ml) coconut oil

1 lb (450 g) fresh or frozen mixed berries, such as raspberries, blueberries, and blackberries

berry jelly

½ cup (55 g) frozen mixed berries

⅓ cup (115 g) raw honey

Juice of ½ lemon

1 tsp unflavoured gelatine powder

to serve

Whipped coconut cream (page 210)

Fresh mixed berries

Fresh baby mint leaves (optional)

To make the crumble, combine the almonds, coconut, vanilla bean seeds, and a pinch of sea salt in a food processor, and process until broken up into a nice crumble. Add the dates and pulse until the mixture just comes together (if you overprocess, the mixture will become oily). Transfer the crumble to a bowl and set aside.

To make the cheesecake, combine the cashews, lime juice, honey, vanilla seeds, and 1 tsp salt in a food processor and process until the mixture is smooth and creamy. Add the coconut oil and process until combined. Add the mixed berries and pulse a few times to mix the berries through.

Divide the crumble among six to eight small glasses, then pour the cheesecake over the crumble, dividing it evenly, and refrigerate for 2 to 3 hours, or until set.

Meanwhile, to make the jelly, combine 1 cup (250 ml) water, the mixed berries, honey, and lemon juice in a small saucepan and bring to a boil. Reduce the heat and simmer until the berries soften, about 5 minutes. Strain the liquid, discarding the berries. In a small bowl, sprinkle the gelatine powder over 2 tbsp water and soak for 2 minutes. Stir the gelatine mixture into the hot berry liquid to dissolve, then strain into a bowl. Let cool completely, then pour over the set cheesecakes, dividing evenly. Refrigerate for 1½ hours or until the jelly is set.

To serve, top each cheesecake with a dollop of whipped coconut cream, then add some mixed berries, and garnish with mint, if using.

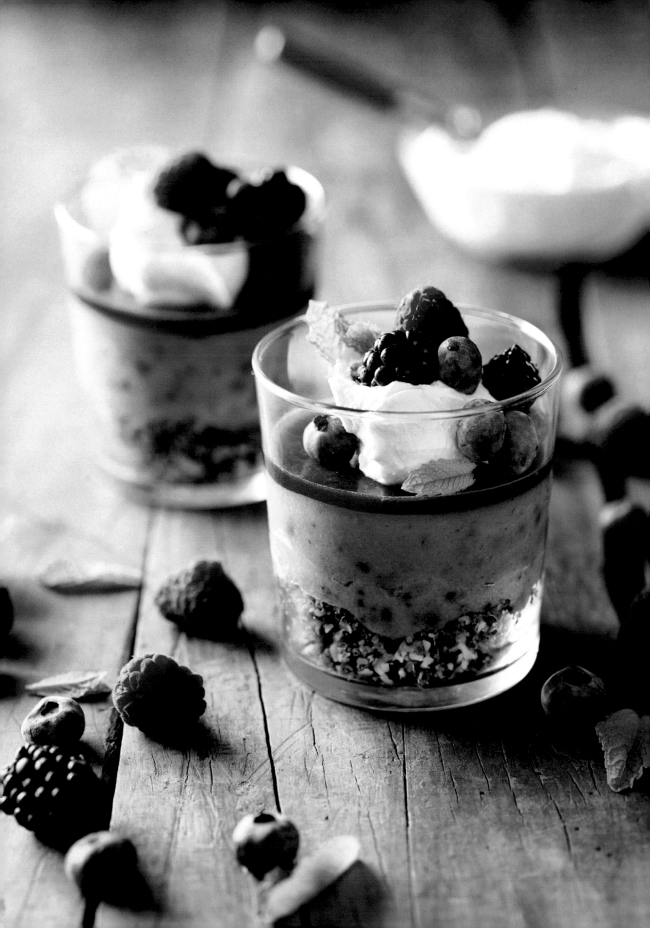

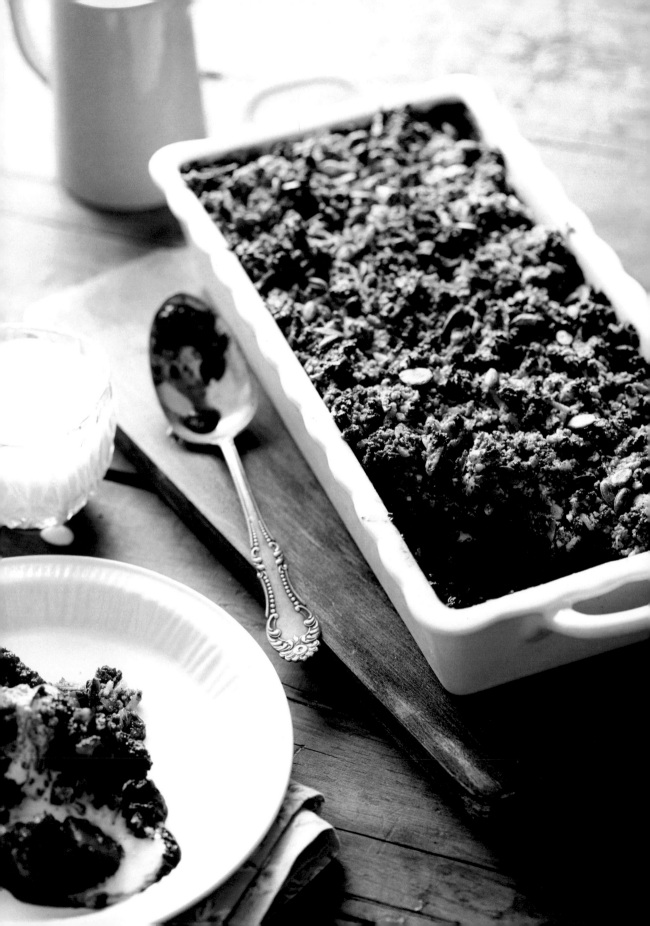

A quintessential crumble is a must for everyone's dessert repertoire. The beauty of this traditional dessert is that you can change it to suit your taste and the seasons. I love this apple and berry version because I can usually get my hands on tart green apples throughout the year, and we always have organic frozen berries in our freezer. It's a wonderful warm dessert to enjoy during the winter months and a lovely refreshing treat to serve chilled during the summer months.

APPLE-BERRY CRUMBLE

SERVES 6

filling
4 apples, peeled, cored, and chopped

¼ cup (85 g) raw honey

1 tbsp coconut oil

Finely grated zest of 1 orange

1 tsp ground cinnamon

1 vanilla bean, split lengthwise and scraped

1½ cups (320 g) fresh or frozen mixed berries

crumble topping
1 cup (100 g) ground almonds or hazelnuts

½ cup (65 g) macadamia nuts, activated (page 209) and finely chopped

½ cup (60 g) pistachio nuts, activated (page 209) and finely chopped

½ cup (40 g) unsweetened shredded dried coconut

6 tbsp (80 g) ghee or coconut oil, at room temperature

¼ cup (85 g) raw honey

½ tsp ground cinnamon

Whipped coconut cream (page 210) or Paleo vanilla ice cream (page 210), to serve

To make the filling, combine the apples, honey, 3 tbsp water, coconut oil, orange zest, cinnamon, and vanilla bean and seeds in a saucepan. Cover and cook over medium-low heat, stirring occasionally, until the apples soften, about 5 minutes. Add the berries, cover, and cook for another 3 to 4 minutes, until the berries start to burst. Remove the vanilla bean.

Meanwhile, to make the topping, combine the ground almonds, macadamia nuts, pistachio nuts, coconut, ghee, honey, cinnamon, and a pinch of sea salt in a bowl. Mix well to combine; the mixture should resemble coarse crumbs.

Preheat the oven to 325°F (160°C gas 3).

Spread the apple mixture evenly into an 8-inch (20 cm) square baking dish. Sprinkle the crumble mix over the apple mixture to cover.

Bake for 10 to 15 minutes, or until golden brown. Remove from the oven and allow to stand for 2 to 3 minutes before serving. Serve with coconut cream or ice cream.

Between the ages of four and eight, my eldest daughter, Chilli, decided that she couldn't stand avocado, but a carob version of this chocolate-avocado mousse was the turning point for her; it made her realize that avocado wasn't all that bad. She now enjoys avocado regularly in all sorts of preparations, from rice-free sushi to smoothies. We choose to use carob in desserts for the kids due to the stimulating nature of cacao. This is a divine dessert to serve on a hot day; its silky smooth texture and chilled temperature is reviving and comforting all blended into one.

CHOCOLATE-AVOCADO MOUSSE
SERVES 4

2 ripe avocados, halved, pitted, and peeled

⅓ cup (40 g) raw cacao or carob powder

2 tbsp raw honey

4 medjool dates, pitted and soaked in warm water for 20 minutes, then drained

1 tsp ground cinnamon

1 vanilla bean, split lengthwise and scraped

8 fresh cherries

Pistachio nuts, activated (page 209)

Toasted coconut shavings, to serve

Combine the avocado, cacao, honey, dates, cinnamon, and vanilla bean seeds in a food processor and blend until very smooth and fluffy.

Spoon the mousse into four small glasses and top each with two cherries, pistachio nuts, and toasted coconut.

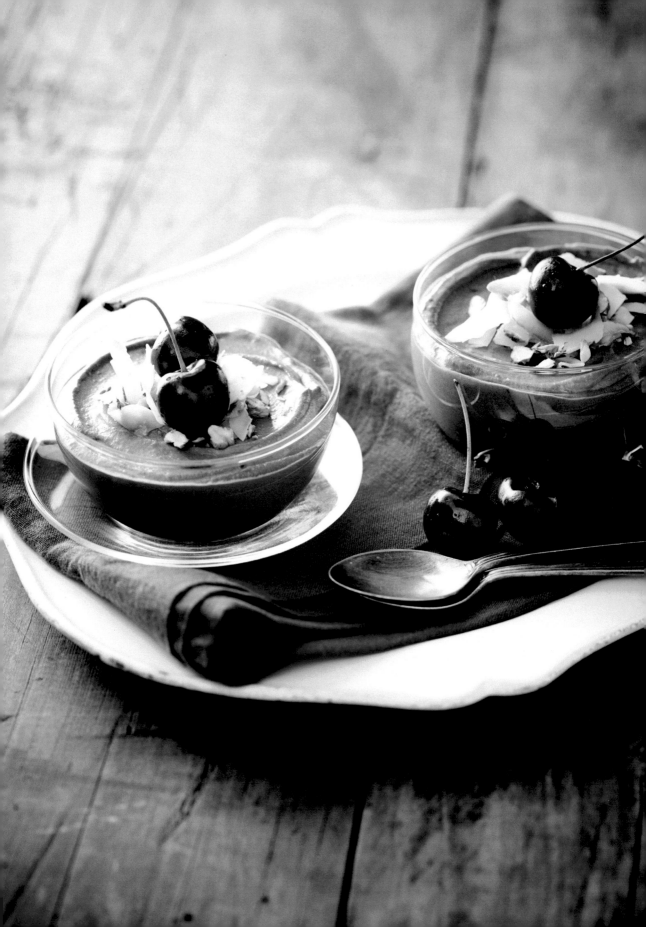

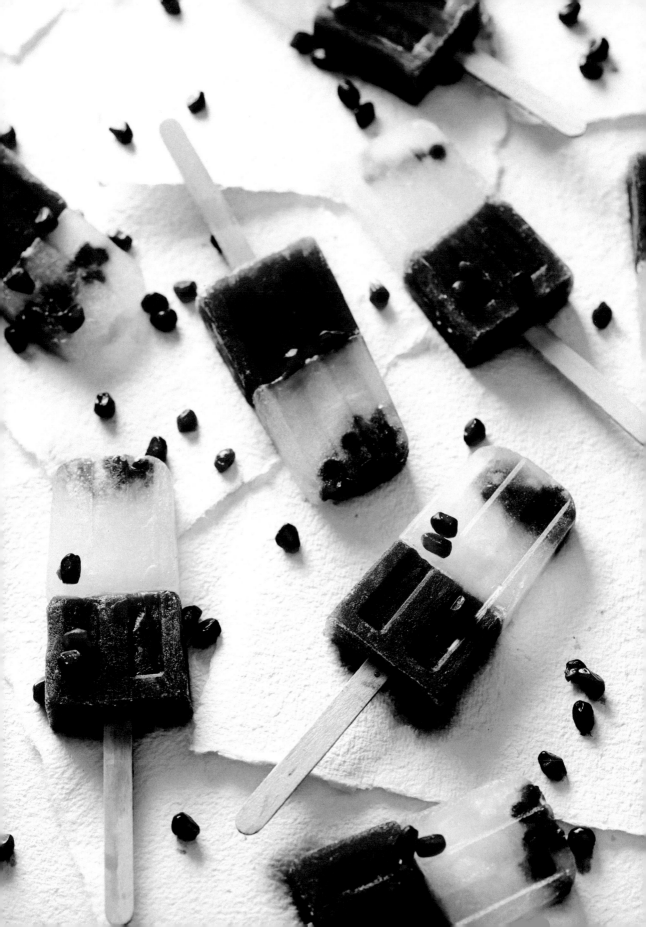

In my younger years, ice lollies were my favourite treat on hot summer days, but shop-bought versions are generally way too high in sugar and unnecessary ingredients. These little treats are just as refreshingly delicious, but they're pure and simple, and my family and I love them. With a little practice, you will master opening fresh coconuts to use their refreshing water and creamy flesh in loads of different ways. In this recipe, I use tart pomegranate juice (easily balanced out with a touch of honey or maple syrup) because I love the flavour and pomegranates' immunity-boosting, digestion-aiding, and antioxidant-rich health benefits. If pomegranates aren't available, use kiwifruit or berries, which work just as well.

POMEGRANATE & COCONUT POPSICLES

SERVES 8

3 pomegranates, halved   1 young green coconut   1 tbsp raw honey, or to taste

Remove 3 tbsp of seeds from one of the pomegranate halves and set aside.

Open the coconut by cutting a circular hole in the top. Pour the coconut water into a measuring cup; you should get about 1 cup (250 ml). Pour the coconut water into eight popsicle moulds so they are half full. Reserve the coconut flesh for another use.

Add a few pomegranate seeds to each mould and freeze for 1 hour. Insert a popsicle stick into each mould, return to the freezer, and freeze for another hour.

Using a non-electric citrus juicer, squeeze and press the pomegranate halves in a circular motion until no more juice is released.

Line a colander with muslin and strain the pomegranate juice; you should get about ½ cup (125 ml) of juice from each pomegranate. Stir in the honey until incorporated. Add more honey to taste, if desired.

Pour the pomegranate juice into the popsicle moulds, and return to the freezer for at least 4 hours, or until frozen.

Note: When buying pomegranates, choose ones that are heavy. They should contain the most juice.

I honestly don't know many people who would turn down the offer of a brownie. This version will dazzle your palate and is sure to fulfill any nagging hankering for chocolate. On special occasions, we like to serve them with a side of homemade coconut ice cream or some raspberry coulis and fresh, juicy berries.

CHOCOLATE BROWNIES

SERVES 6 TO 8

1¼ cups (200 g) raw cacao chocolate (page 210), chopped

¾ cup (185 g) ghee or coconut oil

¼ cup (30 g) raw cacao powder, plus 2 tbsp to dust

6 eggs, separated

¾ cup (250 g) raw honey

2 cups (200 g) walnuts, activated (page 209), toasted, and coarsely chopped

Preheat the oven to 325°F (160°C gas 3). Grease a 7 by 11 by 2-inch (18 by 28 by 5 cm) baking tin, then line with a piece of baking parchment.

Combine the raw cacao chocolate, ghee, and cacao powder in a heatproof bowl set over a saucepan of simmering water (make sure the water isn't touching the bowl); stir occasionally with a spatula until melted and smooth. Remove from the heat and set aside to cool slightly.

Meanwhile, combine the egg yolks and ½ cup (165 g) of the honey in the bowl of a stand mixer fitted with a whisk attachment, and beat at high speed until the mixture doubles in size and is fluffy. Fold the egg mixture into the chocolate until incorporated.

Thoroughly wash and dry the mixing bowl and whisk attachment. Add the egg whites to the bowl along with the remaining ¼ cup (85 g) honey. Beat at high speed until soft peaks form. Fold the egg-white mixture into the chocolate mixture until combined, then gently fold in the walnuts. Pour the mixture into the prepared baking tin and level the top with a palette knife.

Bake for 30 minutes, or until a skewer inserted in the centre comes out clean. The brownie will puff up a little during cooking. Allow to cool, then refrigerate for 2 hours before cutting.

Turn out the brownie onto a cutting board and cut into portions. Dust with extra cacao powder and serve.

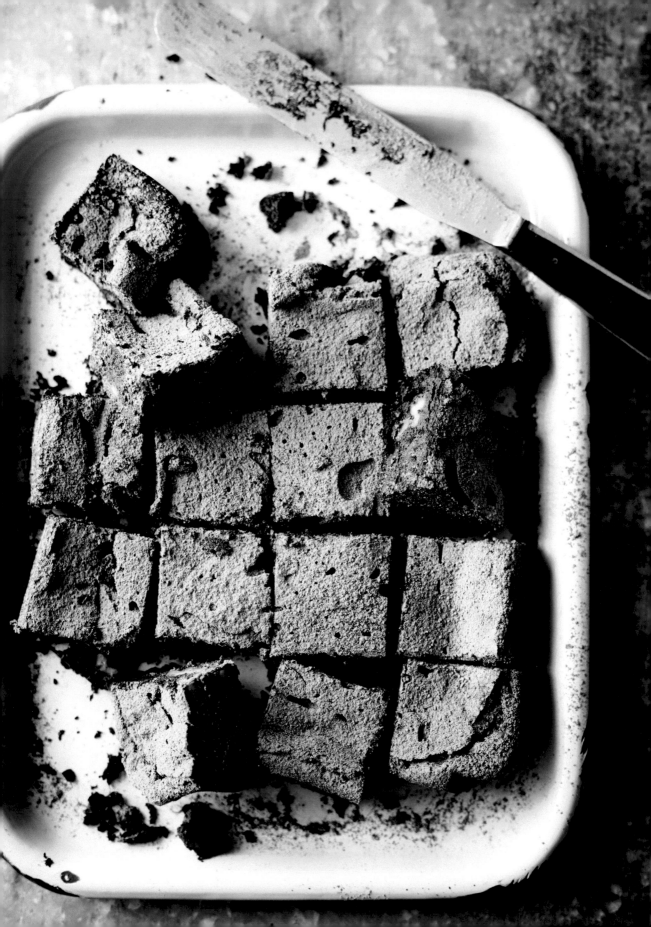

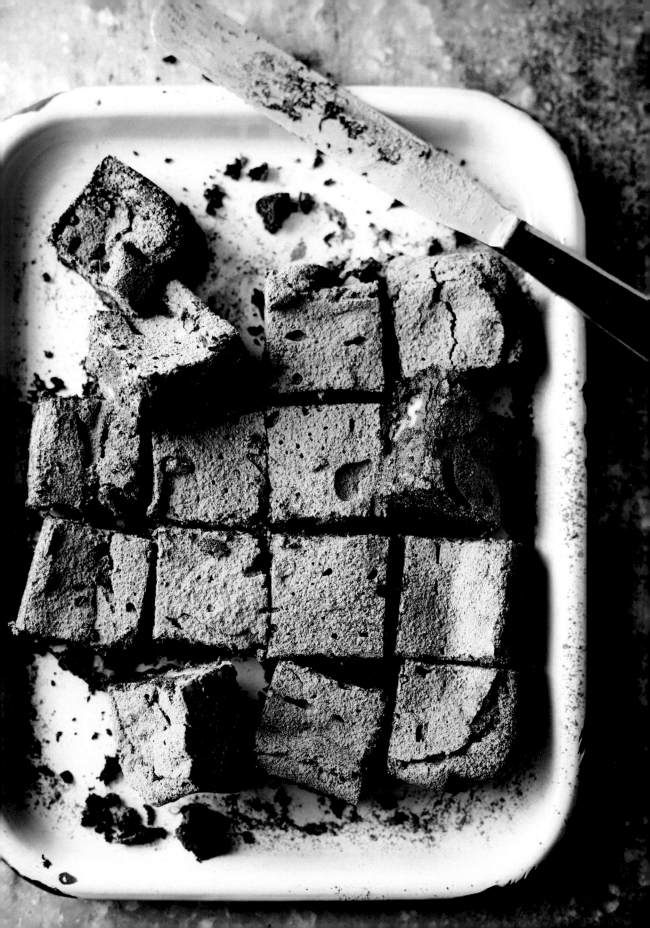

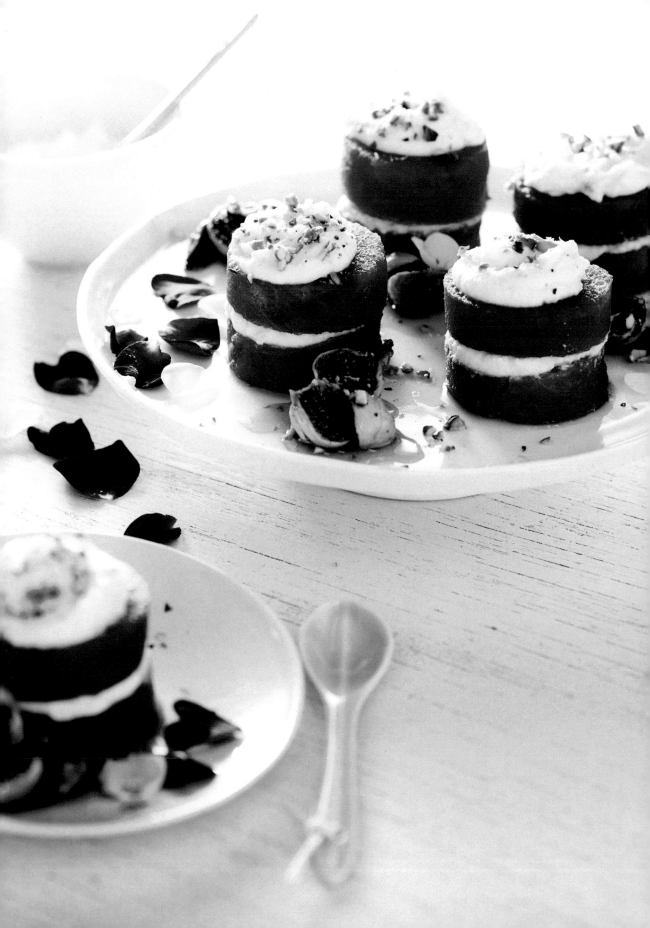

I love these little watermelon cakes on a hot summer day when you feel like something refreshing. Even though they're not really cakes, I do love the shape and the play on words. You can flavour them with whatever you like – watermelon works nicely with both savoury and sweet – but here I have added some of my favourite flavours and ingredients, like rose water-poached figs, creamy coconut, and gorgeous pistachios, to turn it into a delicate but delicious dessert.

WATERMELON 'CAKES'
WITH COCONUT CREAM & ROSE WATER-POACHED FIGS
SERVES 6

poached figs
2 tbsp organic rose water

1 tbsp raw honey

2 cardamom pods, crushed

7 dried baby figs, halved

⅓ cup (100 g) Coconut Vanilla Yoghurt (page 17)

1 cup (190 g) whipped coconut cream (page 210)

¼ seedless watermelon, rind removed and flesh cut into ¾-inch (2 cm) thick slices

¼ cup (30 g) pistachio nuts, activated (page 209) and chopped

To make the poached figs, combine ⅔ cup (150 ml) water, the rose water, honey, and cardamom pods in a small saucepan and bring to a boil over medium-high heat. Add the figs, remove from the heat, cover, and allow to cool completely.

Meanwhile, in a bowl, fold the yoghurt and coconut cream together until blended. Cover and refrigerate for 30 minutes to set.

Cut the watermelon into discs with a 2⅓-inch (6 cm) round cookie cutter; you should have 12 discs.

Lay half the watermelon rounds on six individual dessert plates or a serving platter. Evenly spread about 1 tsp of the chilled yoghurt mixture on each, using half of the mixture. Top each with another round slice on top to form a sandwich and spread another 1 tsp of the yoghurt mixture evenly on each, using the remainder of the mixture and dividing it evenly. Garnish the watermelon cakes with the pistachio nuts and poached figs, then drizzle with some of the syrup. Serve immediately.

Mark Sisson is something of a legend in the Paleo/primal community. He has been a positive guide for countless keen primal followers, and he's renowned for being full of vim and vigour. I'm extremely honoured to be able to share Mark's chocolate bark because it is nothing short of super yummy, and it's certainly a treat that will fully satiate your chocolate desires.

MARK SISSON'S CHOCOLATE BARK
MAKES 12 TO 15 SERVINGS

¾ cup (130 g) raw cacao chocolate (page 210)

1 cup (135 g) macadamia nuts, activated (page 209) and coarsely chopped

½ cup (45 g) unsweetened shredded dried coconut

Line a baking sheet with baking parchment.

Melt the raw cacao chocolate in a heatproof bowl set over a small saucepan filled with 2 inches (5 cm) of simmering water (make the sure water isn't touching the bowl) over medium heat. Stir until smooth.

Mix the macadamia nuts and coconut in a bowl and then spread evenly on the prepared baking sheet. Pour the melted chocolate over the nut mixture and sprinkle sea salt over the chocolate to form a thin even layer. Refrigerate for 2 hours, or until hardened.

Cut or break up into portions to serve. The bark can be stored in an airtight container in the fridge for 1 week, or frozen for up to 2 months.

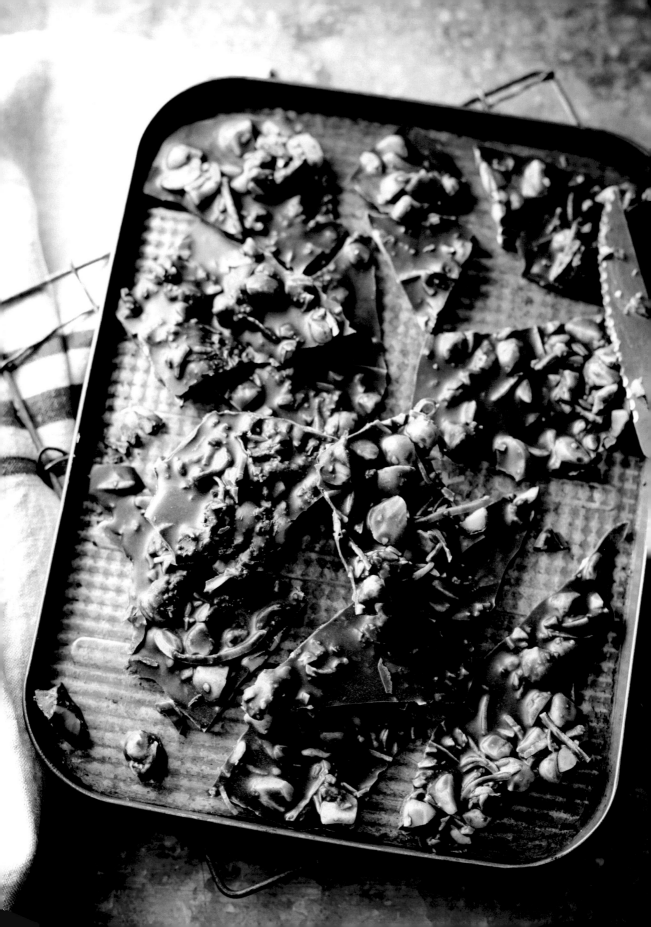

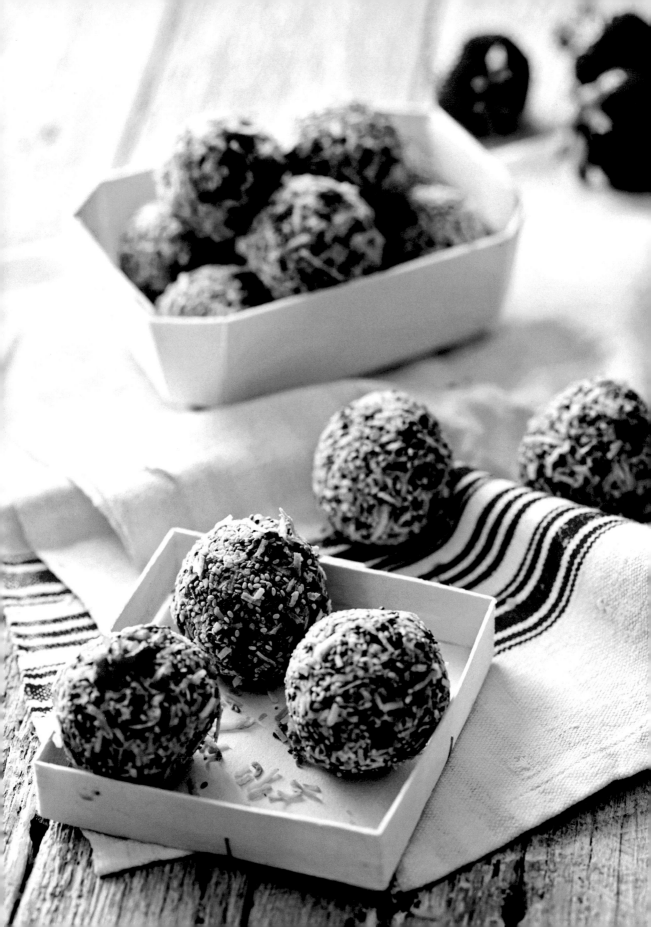

Bliss balls are a regular treat in our house because they're so quick and easy to whip up. You can increase the amount of nuts or seeds and decrease the amount of dried fruit for a less sweet version. They're ideal for school lunches, and little hands make short work in the kitchen, so bliss balls are a wonderful way to get your kids involved in preparing food. My girls love these strawberry bliss balls, so I've chosen this recipe to share with you, but you can add your own personal touch by substituting your favourite dried fruits, nuts, or seeds.

STRAWBERRY BLISS BALLS
MAKES 18

8 medjool dates

¼ banana

1 cup (100 g) walnuts, activated (page 209)

1 cup (135 g) macadamia nuts, activated (page 209) and toasted

3 tbsp coconut oil, melted

⅔ cup (115 g) hulled and chopped strawberries

3 tbsp chia seeds

½ cup (40 g) unsweetened shredded dried coconut, plus extra for rolling

Process the dates in the food processor until smooth. Add the banana, walnuts, macadamia nuts, coconut oil, strawberries, chia seeds, and shredded coconut. Pulse a few times until the mixture just comes together and the nuts have broken down into a crumb-like consistency but still have some texture.

Take a tbsp of the mixture in your hands and roll into a walnut-size ball. Roll the ball in shredded coconut and set on a plate. Repeat until all of the mixture has been formed into small balls. Refrigerate to set for 20 minutes before serving. Store in the refrigerator for up to 1 week.

Pumpkin pie is a symbol of harvest and celebration, so I had to come up with a Paleo version that was as good as the original. I have used a Paleo sweet crust and filled it with dairy-free "custard" that contains tahini and the texture of nuts and seeds. As an added treat, I have included chocolate bacon bark, which has to be tried to be believed.

PUMPKIN PIE
WITH BACON BARK

SERVES 6

Sweet pastry
(page 210), chilled

1 pumpkin, about 1½ lb
(800 g), fibre and seeds removed,
flesh cut into wedges

½ cup (80 g) almonds,
activated (page 209)

½ cup (70 g) Brazil nuts,
activated (page 209)

3 eggs plus 1 egg yolk

½ cup (170 g) raw honey

½ cup (125 ml) coconut milk

1 tbsp unhulled tahini paste

1 tsp ground cinnamon

1 tsp ground ginger

1 tsp freshly grated nutmeg

Whipped coconut cream
(page 210), to serve

Bacon bark (page 210), to serve

Preheat the oven to 350°F (170°C gas 3). Place a large piece of plastic wrap or baking parchment on a work surface. Place the dough on top and roll it out into a 12 inch (30 cm) round, about ¼ inch (5 mm) thick. The dough may crack slightly; don't panic, simply bind it together by pinching it with your fingers and lightly smooth out where the cracks have formed.

Lightly oil a 9-inch (23 cm) pie tin. Place the pie tin upside down on top of the centre of the pastry. Wrap the edges of the plastic or paper around the pan, and gently flip the pastry and the tin over. Press and smooth the pastry firmly into place, ensuring that there are no gaps between the pastry and the pan. Remove the plastic wrap or paper, fix any cracks by pressing the dough together with your fingers, and trim the edges with a knife.

Partially bake the pie shell for 5 minutes, or until the pastry just starts to turn golden (try not to get too much colour on the pastry because you will be baking it again with the pumpkin filling). Set aside to cool in the tin.

To make the pumpkin puree, place the pumpkin wedges on a baking sheet and roast for 30 to 40 minutes, or until soft. Scoop out 1¾ cups (410 ml) pumpkin flesh. Combine the pumpkin flesh and 2 tbsp water in a food processor and process until smooth. (Freeze any remaining roasted pumpkin or use for another recipe.) Remove from the food processor and set aside. Wipe out the food processor bowl.

Combine the almonds and Brazil nuts in the food processor and blend until they have the consistency of fine crumbs. Add the eggs and egg yolk, honey, coconut milk, and tahini and blend for another 2 to 3 minutes until very smooth. Mix in a little cold water, if necessary, to form a smooth puree. Add the pumpkin puree, cinnamon, ginger, nutmeg, and a pinch of sea salt and blend until well combined.

Pour the pumpkin filling into the pie shell and smooth over the top with a palette knife. Bake for 40 to 45 minutes, or until set. If the edges of the pie start to become too brown before the pie is done, cover the edges with aluminium foil and continue baking until the filling is firm. Allow the pie to cool completely in the refrigerator before serving.

To serve, cut into wedges and top with whipped coconut cream and bacon bark.

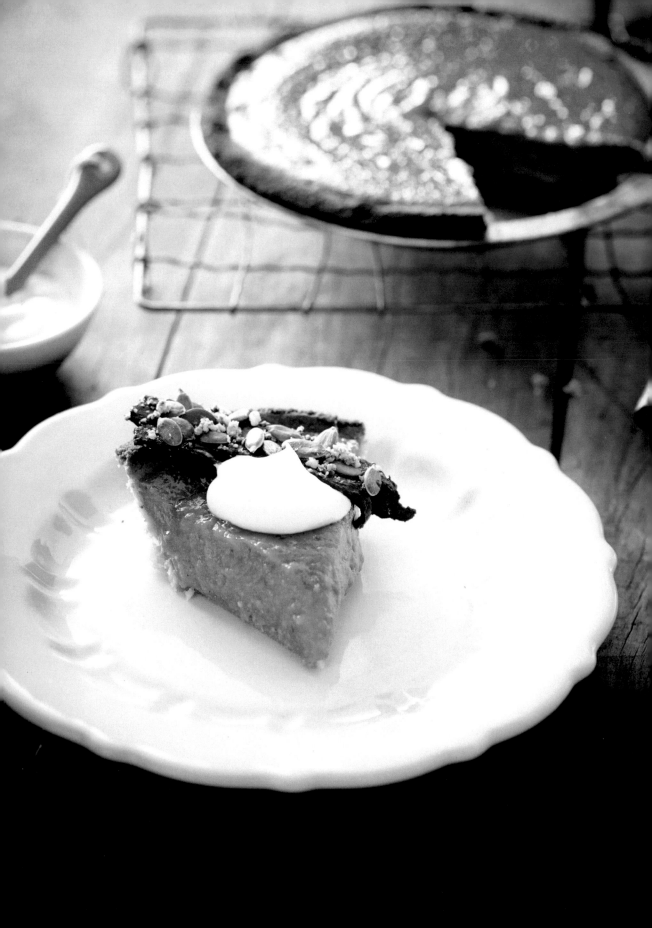

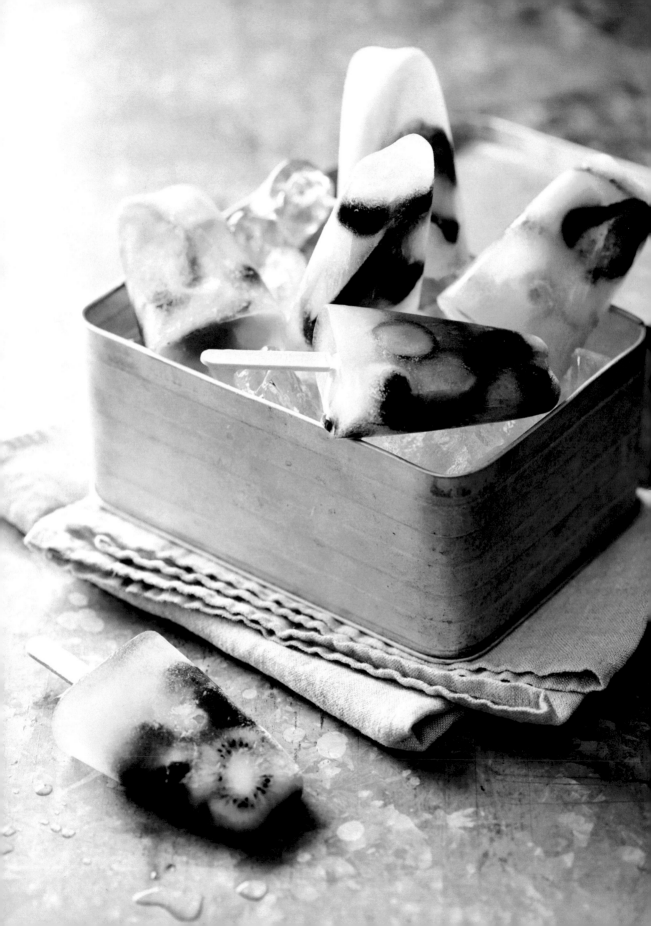

I still remember the instantly refreshing sense you get from sucking on an ice-cold popsicle on a hot summer day, so I just had to include an energizing ice pop that you and your family can make easily at home. It takes almost no time at all to prepare, but make them ahead of time, or you'll have pop-hungry munchkins hanging around the freezer waiting for the pops to freeze. Some of our favourite fruits to use are antioxidant-rich berries, refreshing watermelon, and mangos with a squeeze of lime juice. Try to choose the best-quality, organic, seasonal fruit, free from potentially toxic pesticides; even better, seek out wild or heirloom varieties.

FRUITY ICE POPS

SERVES 8

2 young green coconuts

About 2 cups mixed fresh fruits, such as strawberries, grapes, mangos, lychees, kiwi, raspberries, or pineapple, cut into bite-sized pieces

Open the coconuts by cutting a circular hole in the top of each one. Pour the coconut water into a jug and set aside. Reserve the flesh for another use.

Arrange pieces of fruit in each of eight popsicle moulds, filling the moulds and making sure the pieces fit snugly in the moulds. Pour enough coconut water into each mould to just cover the fruit. Insert popsicle sticks and freeze until solid, at least 6 hours. The popsicles will keep in the freezer for up to 2 weeks.

Anyone who has visited Spain has to admit their churros (doughnuts) are very addictive, especially when served with warm chocolate dipping sauce. I have created a healthy Paleo version here, without using refined sugars or grains, and it is simply divine. If you like, substitute carob for the chocolate in the sauce, particularly if serving this to kids.

CHURROS
WITH CHOCOLATE SAUCE
MAKES 12

7 tbsp (100 g) ghee

1½ tsp raw honey

3½ tbsp (35 g) coconut flour

½ cup (65 g) arrowroot powder

3 eggs

Coconut oil, for deep-frying

Chocolate sauce (page 210), warmed to serve

To make the churros, combine ½ cup (125 ml) water, the ghee, honey, and ¼ tsp sea salt in a saucepan over medium heat and bring to a simmer. Add the coconut flour and arrowroot and stir constantly with a wooden spoon until a ball is formed, about 30 seconds. Continue to stir for another 30 seconds, until the dough comes away from the sides of the pan.

Transfer the dough to the bowl of a stand mixer fitted with a paddle attachment. With the speed set on medium-low, add the eggs, one at a time, and continue to mix for 4 minutes, or until the dough has cooled. Spoon the dough into a piping bag fitted with a ½-inch (13 mm) star tip.

In a deep saucepan, heat the coconut oil to 320°F (160°C); the oil should be about 4 inches (10 cm) deep.

Carefully pipe the churros dough into the hot oil in lengths of about 2¾ inches (7 cm). (You can use a pair of scissors to cut off the dough.) Fry the churros in batches until golden, 1 to 2 minutes. Remove the churros from the oil and place on paper towels to soak up any excess oil.

Serve the churros hot with the chocolate sauce on the side for dipping.

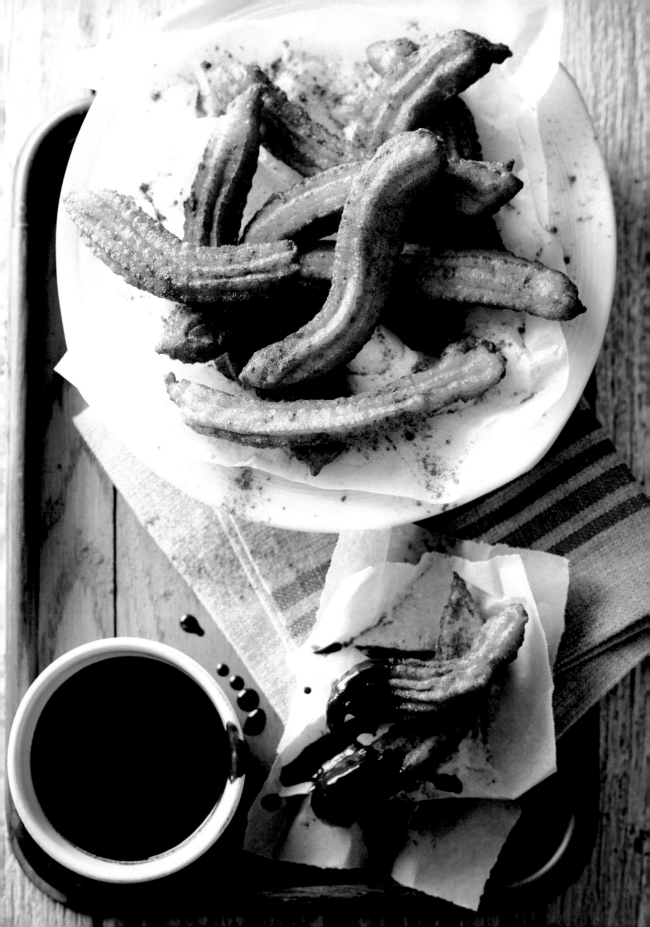

DRINKS

192	196
ginger & liquorice iced tea	green goodness smoothie
192	199
nut milk	green juice
195	199
chai smoothie	beetroot, carrot & kale juice
195	200
hot carob	iced chocolate
196	200
super berry smoothie	chocolate smoothie

GINGER & LIQUORICE ICED TEA

SERVES 2 TO 4

4 liquorice root sticks, broken into pieces

1-inch (2.5 cm) piece fresh ginger, sliced

1 cinnamon stick

2 tbsp raw honey (optional)

½ bunch of mint

Put the liquorice root, ginger, and cinnamon stick in a large heat-resistant container and pour in 4¼ cups (1 L) boiling water. Allow to steep for 20 minutes.

Pour the tea through a clean strainer into a jug, stir, taste, and add the honey, if using, and mint. Let cool to room temperature, then chill in the refrigerator. Strain through a fine sieve, and serve with ice.

NUT MILK

MAKES 1 QUART (1 L)

1 cup (150 g) almonds or other nuts, such as macadamia nuts or walnuts, activated (page 209)

Combine the nuts and 4 cups (1 L) water in a blender and blend for 2 minutes or until smooth.

Line a bowl with a piece of muslin so that the muslin hangs over the edges of the bowl. Pour the blended nuts and water into the bowl. Pick up the edges of the muslin and squeeze out all the milk.

Pour the nut milk into a 1-quart (1 L) jar, place in the refrigerator, and give it a good shake when you want to use it. The nut milk will last for 4 to 5 days.

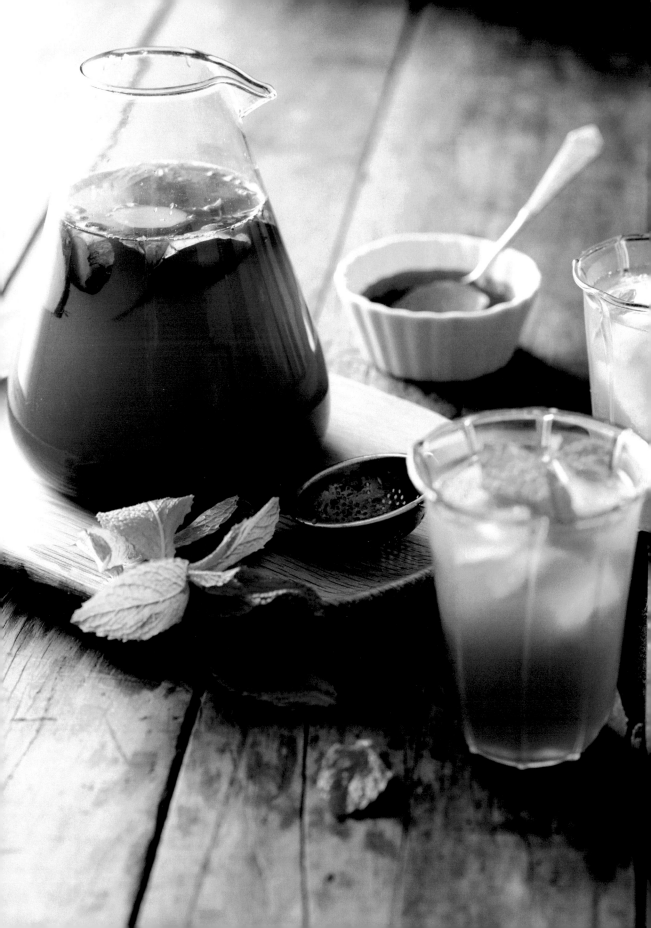

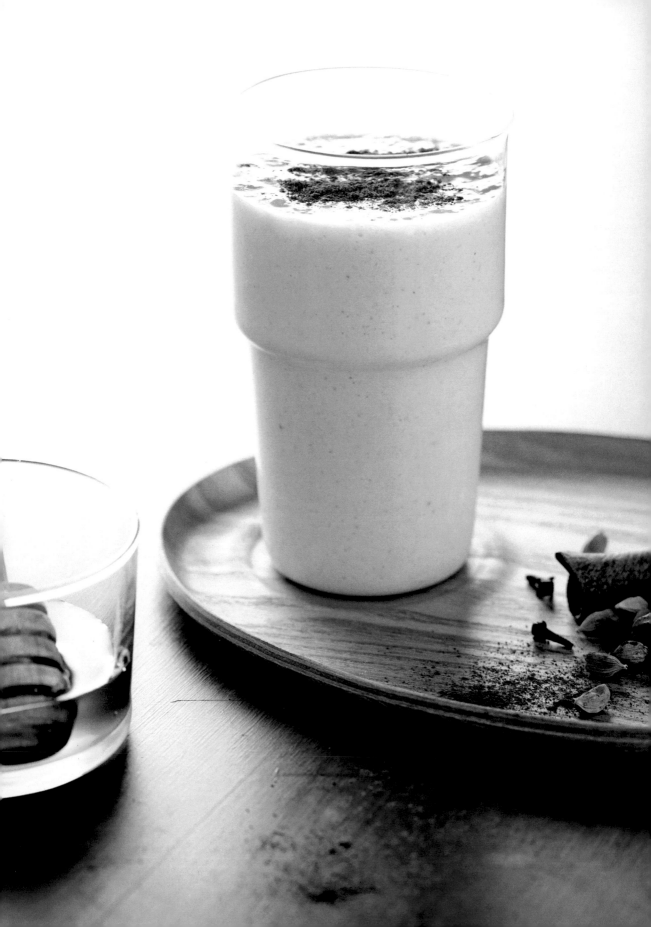

CHAI SMOOTHIE

SERVES 1 TO 2

1 cup (250 ml) coconut water

1 cup (250 ml) coconut cream or coconut milk

2 eggs

1 to 2 bananas, frozen

1 tbsp liquorice root powder (optional; see Note page 196)

1 tbsp raw honey (optional)

1 tsp peeled and finely grated fresh ginger

1 tsp ground cinnamon

½ tsp ground cardamom

½ tsp ground cloves

Combine all the ingredients in a blender and blend until smooth and creamy. Pour into one or two glasses and serve immediately.

Note: You can easily freeze this and turn it into ice cream.

HOT CAROB

SERVES 2

2 cups (500 ml) coconut milk or almond milk (page 192)

2 tbsp carob powder or raw cacao powder (see Note below)

2 tbsp raw honey (optional)

1 pinch ground cinnamon

Vanilla marshmallows (page 211), to serve

Pour the coconut milk into a small saucepan. Whisk in the carob powder, honey, if using, and cinnamon to smooth any lumps. Place the saucepan over medium heat and bring to a simmer, then remove from the stove. Pour the hot carob into mugs, serve with marshmallows if you like, and sit back, take a sip, and enjoy.

Note: Add a little raw cacao powder to give this drink antioxidant benefits. Just be careful how much cacao you give your little ones, because it's a stimulant.

SUPER BERRY SMOOTHIE

SERVES 2

1 tsp spirulina powder

1 cup (160 g) fresh or frozen blueberries

½ cup (60 g) fresh or frozen raspberries

¼ cup (60 g) frozen acai berry pulp, or fresh, if available

1 fresh or frozen banana

1 tbsp raw honey (optional)

½ cup (125 ml) coconut milk or almond milk (page 192)

½ cup (125 ml) coconut water

Flesh of 1 young green coconut (see recipe below)

5 almonds, activated (page 209)

5 macadamia nuts, activated (page 209)

Ice (optional)

Combine all the ingredients in a blender, adding ice if you are using fresh berries. Blend until smooth and creamy. Pour into two tall glasses and serve immediately.

GREEN GOODNESS SMOOTHIE

SERVES 2 TO 3

1 young green coconut

2 eggs

1 cup (160 g) almonds, activated (page 209)

2 cucumbers, chopped

1 to 2 handfuls of spinach

1 bunch of flat-leaf parsley

1 handful of mint leaves

2 tsp ground cinnamon

2 tbsp maca powder (optional; see Note below)

2 tsp liquorice root powder (optional; see Note below)

Open the coconut by cutting a circular hole in the top. Pour the coconut water into a jug; you should get about 1 cup (250 ml). Use a spoon to scoop the flesh out of the coconut; you should get about ¾ cup (120 g). Place in the fridge until needed.

Put the reserved coconut water and flesh in a blender along with 1 cup (250 ml) water, the eggs, almonds, cucumbers, spinach, parsley, mint, cinnamon, and maca and liquorice root, if using. Blend until smooth and creamy. Pour into two or three tall glasses and serve immediately.

Note: Maca packs a punch so it's wise to start off with smaller amounts to see how your system reacts. We use liquorice root powder for its sweetness, but it's very powerful so check with your health care professional if you have any concerns, and do not use it if you're taking warfarin. You can also add all sorts of other ingredients like hemp seeds or powder, chia seeds, maqui berry, camu camu, aloe vera juice, spirulina, ginger, turmeric, cloves, bee pollen, berries . . . the list goes on and on.

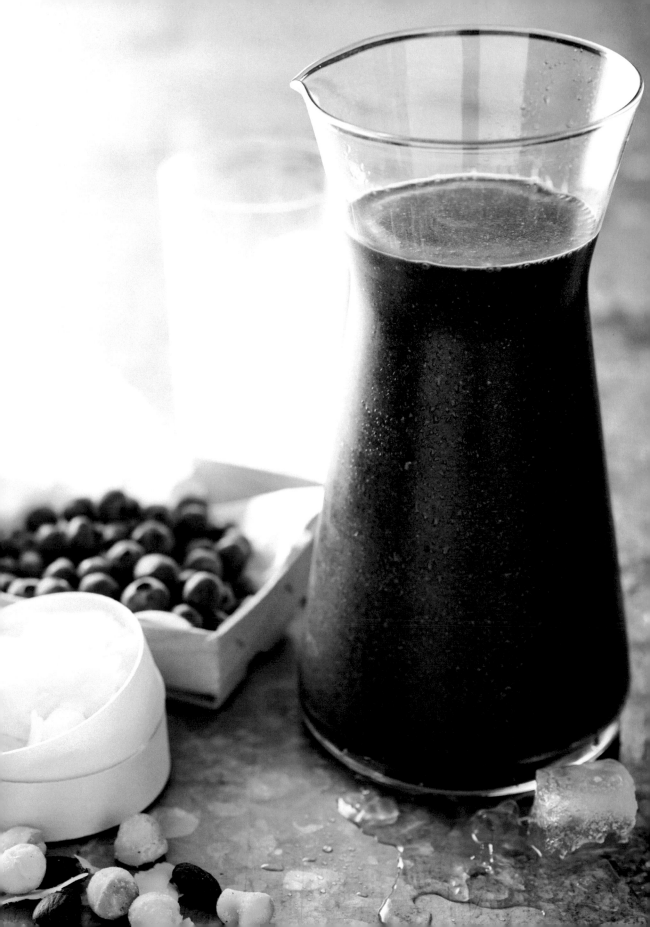

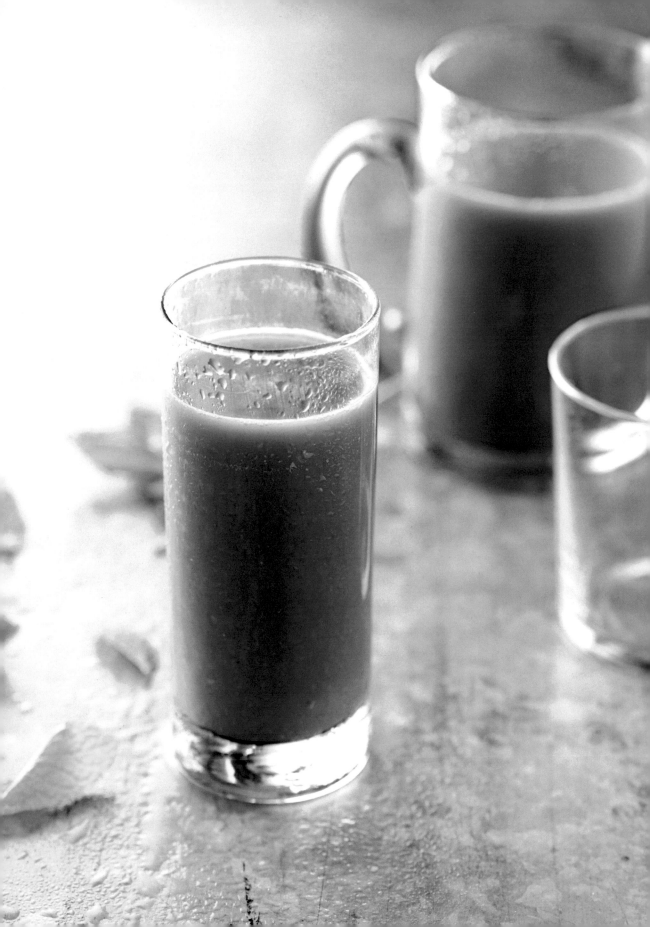

GREEN JUICE

½ bunch of kale

1 handful of spinach

4 celery stalks

2 cucumbers

1 lime, peeled

½ bunch of flat-leaf parsley

½ bunch of mint

4-inch (10 cm) piece fresh ginger

2 green apples

1 tbsp green superfood powder (optional)

Combine all of the ingredients except the superfood powder (if using) in a juicer and juice them together. Stir in the superfood powder. Pour into two tall glasses and serve immediately.

BEETROOT, CARROT & KALE JUICE

2 large beetroots

4 carrots, peeled

2 celery stalks

1 cucumber

1 thumb-size piece fresh ginger

½ bunch of kale

1 orange, peeled

Combine all of the ingredients in a juicer and juice them together. Pour into two glasses and serve immediately.

ICED CHOCOLATE
SERVES 2

2½ cups (600 ml) almond milk (page 192)

1 tbsp raw cacao powder

2 tbsp chocolate sauce (page 210), warmed, plus extra for decorating the glasses

Raw honey, to taste

Ice

2 to 4 scoops Paleo vanilla or chocolate ice cream (page 210)

Whipped coconut cream (page 210), to serve

Finely chopped nuts and/or cacao nibs, to serve (optional)

Combine the almond milk, cacao powder, and chocolate sauce in a blender and blend until smooth (you can add less or more chocolate sauce to your liking). Sweeten to taste with honey if desired.

Pour a little chocolate sauce into two glasses and swirl the glasses around on an angle to get a nice design. Then add a little ice and a couple of scoops of ice cream. Pour in the chocolate milk. Finish with some whipped coconut cream. If you like, dust a little cacao over the top or sprinkle with finely chopped nuts and/or cacao nibs.

CHOCOLATE SMOOTHIE
SERVES 2

2 tbsp raw cacao powder (or carob for children; see Note below)

1 tbsp maca powder (optional; see Note below)

1 tbsp liquorice root powder (optional; see Note below)

½ cup (80 g) fresh or frozen blueberries

1 fresh or frozen banana

2 cups (500 ml) coconut water

½ cup (125 ml) coconut milk or coconut cream

⅓ cup (25 g) shredded coconut

10 almonds, activated (page 209)

10 macadamia nuts, activated (page 209)

1 tbsp raw honey

Ice (optional)

Combine the cacao powder, maca powder (if using), liquorice root powder (if using), blueberries, banana, coconut water, coconut milk, shredded coconut, almonds, macadamia nuts, and honey in a blender and blend until smooth and creamy. If you're using fresh blueberries instead of frozen, add a little ice to the blender, too. Pour into two tall glasses and serve.

Note: If you are making this for your kids, substitute carob for the cacao powder and leave out the maca and liquorice root (for more information on maca and liquorice root, see page 196).

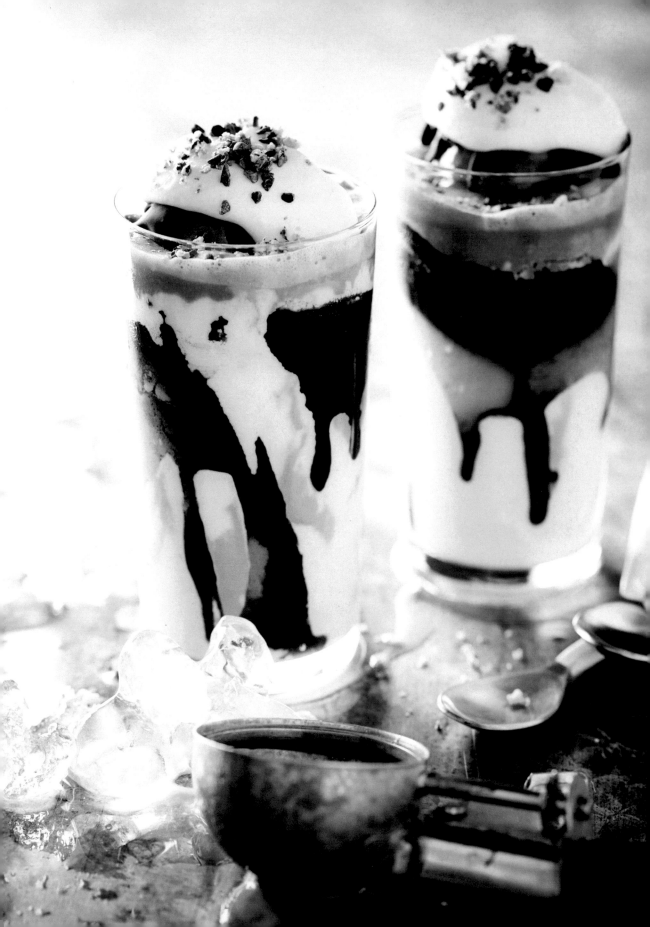

BASICS

VEGETABLE STOCK

MAKES ABOUT 3½ QT (3.25 L)

1 tbsp coconut oil

1 onion, coarsely chopped

2 large carrots, peeled and coarsely chopped

2 parsnips, peeled and coarsely chopped

1 celery stalk, coarsely chopped

½ bunch of Swiss chard, stems and leaves roughly chopped

2 to 3 sprigs thyme

2 to 3 fresh flat-leaf parsley stems

1 dried or fresh bay leaf

In a stockpot or large saucepan over medium-high heat, melt the oil. Add the onion and cook, stirring, until caramelized, about 8 minutes. Add the carrots, parsnips, and celery and cook until tender, about 15 minutes.

Add 4¼ qt (4 L) water, the Swiss chard, thyme, parsley, and bay leaf. Bring to a boil, reduce the heat to low, and simmer until the stock is highly flavoured, about 1 hour.

Remove the stock from the heat and strain through a fine-mesh sieve into storage containers, pressing on the vegetables to extract all their juices. Discard the vegetables. The stock can be refrigerated for 3 to 4 days or frozen for up to 3 months.

FISH STOCK

MAKES ABOUT 2½ QT (2.5 L)

2 tbsp coconut oil

2 onions, coarsely chopped

1 carrot, peeled and coarsely chopped

½ cup (125 ml) dry white wine or vermouth (optional)

3 or 4 whole, non-oily fish carcasses (including heads), from fish such as snapper, halibut, cod, or flounder

3 tbsp raw apple cider vinegar

2 to 3 sprigs thyme

2 to 3 fresh flat-leaf parsley stems

1 bay leaf

Melt the oil in a stockpot or large saucepan over medium-low heat. Add the onions and carrot and cook very gently until soft, about 30 minutes. Pour in the wine, if using, and bring to a boil over medium-high heat. Add the fish carcasses and cover with 3¼ qt (3 L) cold water. Stir in the vinegar and bring to a boil,

skimming off any scum and impurities as they rise to the top. Tie the thyme, parsley, and bay leaf together with kitchen string and add to the pot. Reduce the heat to low, cover, and simmer for 2 hours.

Remove the carcasses with tongs or a slotted spoon and strain the liquid into storage containers for the refrigerator or freezer. Chill well in the refrigerator and remove any congealed fat before transferring to the freezer for long-term storage. The fish stock can be stored in the refrigerator for 3 to 4 days or frozen for up to 3 months.

CHICKEN STOCK

MAKES ABOUT 3¼ QT (3 L)

2¼ to 3⅓ lb (1 to 1.5 kg) bony chicken parts, such as necks, backs, breast bones, and wings

2 to 4 chicken feet (optional)

2 tbsp raw apple cider vinegar

1 large onion, coarsely chopped

2 carrots, peeled and coarsely chopped

3 celery stalks, coarsely chopped

2 leeks, white part only, coarsely chopped

1 head garlic, halved crosswise

1 tbsp black peppercorns, lightly crushed

2 large handfuls of fresh flat-leaf parsley stems

Put the chicken parts in a stockpot or large saucepan and add 4¼ qt (4 L) cold water, the vinegar, onion, carrots, celery, leeks, garlic, and peppercorns and let stand for 30 to 60 minutes.

Bring to a boil over medium-high heat, skimming off any scum that forms on the surface of the liquid. Turn down the heat to low and simmer for at least 6 and up to 8 hours. The longer you cook the stock, the richer and more flavourful it will be. About 10 minutes before the stock is ready, add the parsley.

Strain the stock through a fine-mesh sieve into a large storage container, cover, and place in your refrigerator until the fat rises to the top and congeals. Skim off this fat and reserve the stock in covered containers in your refrigerator or freezer. The stock can be stored in the refrigerator for 3 to 4 days or frozen for up to 3 months.

Note: Farm-raised, free-range chickens give the best results. Caged chickens may not produce stock that sets.

BEEF STOCK

MAKES ABOUT 3¼ QT (3 L)

About 2¼ lb (2 kg) beef knuckle and marrow bones

1 calf's foot, cut into pieces (optional)

3 tbsp raw apple cider vinegar

3⅓ lb (1.5 kg) meaty rib or neck bones

3 onions, coarsely chopped

3 carrots, peeled and coarsely chopped

2 leeks, white part only, coarsely chopped

3 celery stalks, coarsely chopped

2 or 3 sprigs thyme, tied together

1 tsp black peppercorns, crushed

1 head garlic, halved crosswise

2 large handfuls of fresh flat-leaf parsley stems

Place the knuckle bones, marrow bones, and calf's foot (if using) in a stockpot or very large saucepan. Add the vinegar and pour in 4¼ qt (4 L) cold water (enough to cover). Let stand for 1 hour.

Preheat the oven to 400°F (200°C gas 6).

Put the meaty rib bones, onions, carrots, and leeks in a roasting tin and roast for 10 minutes, until well browned. Add to the stockpot along with the celery.

Pour the fat out of the roasting tin into a separate saucepan and add 4½ cups (about 1 L) water. Place the saucepan over high heat, and bring to a simmer, stirring with a wooden spoon to loosen any coagulated juices. Add this liquid to the bones and vegetables. Add additional water, if necessary, to cover the bones; the liquid should come no higher than within ¾ inch (2 cm) of the rim of the stockpot because the volume increases slightly during cooking.

Bring the stock to a boil, skimming off any scum that rises to the top. Turn down the heat to low and add the thyme, peppercorns, and garlic.

Simmer the stock for at least 8 hours or up to 12 hours. About 10 minutes before the stock is ready, add the parsley. Strain the stock through a fine-mesh sieve into a large container. Cover and cool in the refrigerator. Remove the congealed fat that rises to the top. Transfer to smaller airtight containers. The stock can be stored in the refrigerator for 3 to 4 days or frozen for up to 3 months.

MAYONNAISE

MAKES ABOUT 1¾ CUPS (415 ML)

1 egg plus 2 egg yolks

2 tbsp raw apple cider vinegar

2 tbsp freshly squeezed lemon juice

1 tsp of fermented mustard (page 206)

1½ cups (350 ml) light olive oil or macadamia nut oil

Combine the egg and egg yolks, vinegar, lemon juice, mustard, and 1 tsp sea salt in a food processor or blender and process for 1 to 2 minutes, until combined. With the food processor or blender running, slowly pour in the oil; the oil will begin to emulsify. Keep pouring slowly and consistently, until the mixture becomes thick and looks like mayonnaise. Refrigerate immediately, for at least 5 minutes before using. Mayonnaise will keep for to 4 to 5 days in the refrigerator.

AÏOLI

MAKES ABOUT 2 CUPS (500 ML)

4 egg yolks

2 tbsp raw apple cider vinegar

2 tbsp freshly squeezed lemon juice

2 tsp fermented mustard (page 206) or Dijon mustard

4 confit garlic cloves (page 207), finely chopped

1¾ cups (400 ml) light olive oil or macadamia nut oil

Combine the egg yolks, vinegar, lemon juice, mustard, and garlic in a bowl and blend with a hand-held stick blender. As you blend, slowly pour in the oil in a thin stream, until the aïoli is thick and creamy. Season with sea salt and freshly cracked black pepper. Cover with plastic wrap and refrigerate until needed. It will keep for 4 to 5 days.

CHIPOTLE AÏOLI

MAKES ABOUT 1¼ CUPS (280 ML)

2 chipotles in adobo sauce, or to taste

1 tbsp adobo sauce

1 cup (250 ml) aïoli or to taste

Combine all the ingredients in a food processor and process until smooth. Add more aïoli if the flavour is too spicy for your liking, or add more chipotles if you prefer it extra spicy. Transfer to an airtight container and store in the refrigerator; it will keep for 4 to 5 days.

ARTICHOKE TARTAR SAUCE

MAKES 1 CUP (250 ML)

½ cup (125 ml) aïoli (page 203)

4 small jarred artichokes hearts, finely chopped

1 tsp finely chopped baby capers

1 tsp finely chopped cornichons

1 tsp finely chopped shallot

1 tsp finely chopped fresh flat-leaf parsley

In a bowl, combine all the ingredients together and mix well. Transfer to an airtight container and store in the refrigerator; it will keep for 4 to 5 days.

GREEN GODDESS DRESSING

MAKES 1 CUP (250 ML)

½ avocado, halved, pitted, and peeled

¼ cup (60 ml) coconut milk

3 tbsp (45 ml) freshly squeezed lemon juice

1 clove garlic, finely chopped

2 salt-packed anchovy fillets, rinsed, dried, and finely chopped

½ cup (30 g) coarsely chopped fresh flat-leaf parsley

¼ cup (10 g) coarsely chopped fresh basil

1 tbsp coarsely chopped fresh tarragon

½ cup (120 ml) extra virgin olive oil

Combine the avocado, coconut milk, lemon juice, garlic, anchovies, parsley, basil, tarragon, and ¼ tsp sea salt in a food processor and process until combined. With the machine running, slowly pour in the oil and process until the dressing thickens and the herbs are finely chopped. Store in the refrigerator for up to 5 days.

ROMESCO SAUCE

MAKES 1¼ CUPS (300 ML)

2 vine-ripened tomatoes, halved

1 fresh red chilli, seeded and cut lengthwise

1 tsp sweet paprika

1 tbsp coconut oil, melted

12 blanched almonds, activated and lightly toasted (page 209)

12 hazelnuts, activated (page 209), and lightly toasted, skins removed

2 roasted red peppers (page 208) seeded

3 cloves garlic, finely chopped

2 tbsp red wine vinegar

⅓ cup (80 ml) extra virgin olive oil

Place the tomato and chilli halves in a bowl and sprinkle with the paprika, then drizzle with the coconut oil. Season with sea salt and freshly cracked black pepper

and toss to coat evenly. Preheat a grill pan over high heat. Place the tomato and chilli halves in the pan, skin side down, and grill until soft and the skins have blistered, about 4 minutes. Peel and coarsely chop.

Combine the almonds and hazelnuts in a food processor and process until finely ground. Add the roasted red peppers, chopped tomatoes and chilli, garlic, and vinegar and process to form a paste. With the machine still running, slowly add the olive oil until well combined. Season with salt and pepper. Transfer to a bowl, cover with plastic wrap, and refrigerate until needed, up to 1 week.

RED CURRY PASTE

MAKES ¾ CUP (200 G)

12 dried long red chillies, seeded (⅓ oz/10 g total)

1½ tbsp coriander seeds

1 tbsp cumin seeds

1 tsp black peppercorns

4 tbsp coconut oil

2 to 3 fresh bird's eye chillies, seeded and chopped

2 tbsp finely chopped shallot

2 tbsp garlic, finely chopped

1 tbsp peeled and grated galangal

2 tbsp finely chopped lemongrass, tender white part only

1 tbsp finely chopped coriander stems

2 tsp shrimp paste

1 kaffir lime leaf, finely chopped

Soak the dried chillies in hot water to cover for 15 minutes, until they soften slightly.

Meanwhile, combine the coriander, cumin, and peppercorns in a dry frying pan and toast the spices over medium heat until fragrant, 2 minutes. Remove from the heat and let cool. Using a large mortar and pestle, grind to a fine powder.

Drain the water from the dried chillies and transfer to the mortar. Pound with the pestle to break down the chillies.

Add the coconut oil to the frying pan over medium heat. When the oil is hot, add the fresh bird's eye chillies, shallot, garlic, galangal, lemongrass, and coriander stems, and cook for 5 minutes, or until soft and fragrant. Transfer to the mortar and add the shrimp paste, lime leaf, and 1 tsp sea salt. Pound to a smooth paste (it is important that the paste be smooth). Alternatively, use a food processor to blend the ingredients, using up to ⅓ cup (80 ml) water while blending to create a smooth paste.

The paste will keep in the refrigerator for up to 1 month.

YELLOW CURRY PASTE

MAKES 1 CUP (250 G)

6 dried hot red chillies

4 tbsp coconut oil

10 cloves garlic, finely chopped

6 shallots, finely chopped

1 tsp shrimp paste

2-inch (5 cm) piece fresh ginger, peeled and grated

1-inch (2.5 cm) piece fresh galangal, peeled and grated

2-inch (5 cm) piece fresh turmeric, peeled and grated

4 kaffir lime leaves, chopped

In a bowl, soak the chillies in 1 cup (250 ml) hot water to cover for 30 minutes. Drain the chillies, reserving ⅓ cup (80 ml) of the soaking liquid.

In a frying pan over medium heat, warm the coconut oil. When the oil is hot, add the chillies, 1 tsp sea salt, and the remaining ingredients. Cook for 5 to 10 minutes, or until the mixture is soft and fragrant. Transfer to a food processor, add the reserved soaking liquid, and blend to a fine paste. Store in a sealed container in the refrigerator for up to 1 month.

HARISSA

MAKES ABOUT 1 CUP (250 ML)

1½ oz (42 g) dried hot red chillies, seeded (wear gloves!)

2 fresh red chillies

½ tsp caraway seeds

¼ tsp coriander seeds

¼ tsp cumin seeds

⅓ cup (80 ml) light olive oil

4 cloves garlic, peeled

2 tbsp freshly squeezed lemon juice

½ tsp tomato paste

Preheat the oven to 400°F (200°C gas 6). Place the dried chillies in a bowl and cover with hot water. Soak for 30 minutes.

Put the fresh chillies on a baking sheet and roast for 20 minutes, or until blistered. Remove from the oven and put in a brown paper bag or wrap in a paper towel to cool. Scrape away the charred skin, remove and discard the seeds, and coarsely chop.

Lightly toast the caraway, coriander, and cumin seeds in a dry frying pan over medium heat until aromatic, about 3 minutes. Grind in a spice grinder or mortar and pestle.

Combine the dried and fresh chillies, toasted spices, olive oil, garlic, lemon juice, tomato paste, and ½ tsp sea salt in a food processor. Pulse until well combined and smooth.

Transfer the harissa to a clean glass preserving jar, seal with the lid, and store in the refrigerator. The harissa will keep for 1 month in the refrigerator.

FERMENTED HOT CHILLI SAUCE

MAKES 4 CUPS (1 L)

1 (2 to 5 g) packet vegetable starter culture (size varies by brand)

2¼ lb (1.5 kg) fresh red chillies

4 to 6 cloves garlic, peeled

2 tbsp raw honey

You will need a 1-quart (1 L) glass preserving jar with an airlock lid for this recipe. Wash the jar and utensils thoroughly in very hot water or run them through the hot rinse cycle in a dishwasher.

Dissolve the starter culture in water according to the packet instructions; the amount of water will depend on the brand that you are using.

Combine the chillies, garlic, honey, 2 tsp salt, and the dissolved starter culture in a food processor and process to a fine paste. Spoon into your preserving jar; seal with the lid fitted with an airlock. Allow to ferment at room temperature (61°F to 73°F/16°C to 23°C) for 5 to 7 days in a dark spot in your pantry. Alternatively, you can store the jar in a portable cooler.

After the chilli paste has bubbled and brewed for about a week, if you would like to remove the seeds, set a fine-mesh sieve over a bowl, pour the fermented chilli paste into the sieve, and press down with a wooden spoon to extract as much chilli sauce as possible. Discard the solids.

Transfer the strained chilli sauce to a sterilized preserving jar, seal with the lid, and store in the refrigerator. The sauce will keep for a few months in the refrigerator.

FERMENTED MUSTARD

MAKES 1 CUP (250 ML)

¾ cup (185 ml) fermented brine liquid, strained from Sauerkraut (page 66)

7 tbsp (80 g) brown and yellow mustard seeds (brown are hotter and will make a spicier mustard)

1 shallot, finely chopped

½ tbsp finely chopped garlic

1 tbsp maple syrup

You will need a ½-pint (250 ml) glass preserving jar with an airlock lid for this recipe. Wash the jar and utensils thoroughly in very hot water or run them through a hot rinse cycle in the dishwasher.

Combine the fermented brine liquid, mustard seeds, shallot, and garlic in a glass or stainless steel bowl and allow to soak at room temperature overnight.

In a food processor, combine the soaked mustard seed mixture with the maple syrup and process until you get a texture you like; this can take several minutes. Taste for salt and correct the seasoning.

Transfer the mustard to a clean jar, seal with the lid, and store in the refrigerator. The mustard will keep for a few months in the refrigerator.

FERMENTED KETCHUP

MAKES ABOUT 3 CUPS (750 ML)

⅓ (2 to 5 g) packet vegetable starter culture (packet sizes vary depending on brand)

2 cups (500 g) tomato paste, preferably homemade

¼ cup (90 g) raw honey or maple syrup

2 tbsp raw apple cider vinegar

1 clove garlic, finely chopped

1 fresh red chilli, halved, seeded, and thinly sliced

1 tsp ground allspice

½ tsp ground cloves

You will need a 1-quart (750 ml) glass preserving jar with an airlock lid for this recipe. Wash the jar and utensils thoroughly in very hot water or run them through a hot rinse cycle in the dishwasher.

Dissolve the starter culture in water according to the packet instructions; the amount of water will depend on the brand that you are using. Spoon the tomato paste into a large glass or stainless steel bowl and fold in the honey. Add the starter culture, ½ cup (120 ml) water, the vinegar, garlic, chilli, allspice, cloves, 1 tsp sea salt, and some freshly cracked black pepper. Continue whisking until smooth and uniform. Add extra water or vinegar if you like a thinner sauce.

Spoon the ketchup into the preserving jar and close with a lid fitted with an airlock to seal. Wrap a towel around the jar to block out any light, leaving the airlock exposed. Place the jar in a dark, warm (60°F to 74°F/16°C to 23°C) spot – or in a portable cooler to maintain a more consistent temperature – and allow to culture for 3 to 5 days. The warmer the weather, the shorter the time it needs to ferment. The longer you leave the jar, the higher the level of good bacteria present. It's up to you how long you leave it to ferment – some people prefer the tangier flavour that results from a longer fermenting time, while others prefer a milder flavour.

Transfer the ketchup to a clean preserving jar, seal with the lid, and store in the refrigerator. The ketchup will keep for a few months in the refrigerator.

TABIL (TUNISIAN SPICE BLEND)

MAKES ¼ CUP (30 G)

¼ cup (20 g) coriander seeds

2 tbsp cumin seeds

1 tbsp caraway seeds

2 tsp red chilli flakes

2 tsp garlic powder

Place the coriander, cumin, caraway, and red chilli flakes in a small frying pan over medium-low heat and toast the spices, swirling the pan constantly, for about 3 minutes, or until lightly golden and fragrant. Remove from the heat and let cool.

Transfer the spice mix to a spice grinder or mortar and pestle and grind to a fine powder. Stir in the garlic powder. Store in an airtight container for up to 1 month.

TURKISH SPICE MIX

MAKES ABOUT 1 CUP (80 G)

6½ tbsp (35 g) ground cumin

3 tbsp dried mint

3 tbsp dried oregano

2 tbsp sweet paprika

2 tbsp freshly cracked black pepper

2 tsp hot paprika

Place all the ingredients in an airtight container and shake to mix well. Store for up to 9 months.

CONFIT GARLIC CLOVES

MAKES 25 CONFIT GARLIC CLOVES

25 cloves garlic, peeled

1 cup (250 ml) coconut oil or macadamia nut oil

Combine the garlic cloves and oil in a saucepan over very low heat (you do not want the oil to boil). Cook for 2 hours, or until the garlic is soft. Let cool completely, then store the garlic confit in the oil in a sealed jar in the fridge. It will last for 2 weeks.

FRIED GARLIC

MAKES 4 TBSP

6 cloves garlic, thinly sliced

1 cup (250 ml) coconut oil, melted

Combine the garlic and coconut oil in a small saucepan and heat over medium heat until the garlic starts to turn golden, 2 to 4 minutes. Keep a close eye on it as it may colour a lot faster depending on how thinly the garlic is sliced. Lift the garlic out with a slotted spoon and drain on paper towels. Store in an airtight container for up to 2 weeks.

FRIED SHALLOTS

MAKES 5 TBSP

4 shallots, thinly sliced

2 cups (500 ml) coconut oil, melted

Combine the shallots and coconut oil in a small saucepan and heat over medium heat until the shallots starts to turn golden, 2 to 4 minutes. Keep a close eye on them as they may colour faster depending on how thinly they are sliced. Lift the shallots out with a slotted spoon and drain on paper towels. Store in an airtight container for up to 2 weeks.

FRIED CHILLIES

MAKE 5 TBSP CHILLIES AND 2 CUPS (500 ML)

4 fresh red chillies, thinly sliced

2 cups (500 ml) coconut oil, melted

Combine the chillies and coconut oil in a small saucepan and heat over medium heat until the chillies start to turn a light golden, 2 to 4 minutes. Lift the chilli slices out with a slotted spoon and drain on paper towels. The chillies can be stored in an airtight container for 1 week. The oil can be used as chilli oil for other recipes.

SEED CRACKERS

SERVES 6 TO 8

1 cup (150 g) golden or brown linseeds

⅔ cup (80 g) mixed seeds, such as pumpkin, sunflower, sesame

1 tsp of your favorite spice, such as cayenne, smoked paprika, ground cumin, or fennel seeds (see below for other variations)

Put the linseeds in a bowl, pour over enough water to cover, and leave overnight. Place the mixed seeds in a separate bowl, pour over enough water to cover, and leave overnight.

The next morning, drain the linseeds and drain and rinse the mixed seeds. Add the mixed seeds to the linseeds, which will have a jelly-like texture. Add the spice and ½ tsp sea salt and transfer to a blender. Pulse a few times to break up the seeds (but do not overpulse; you want the seeds to be chopped but a little chunky).

Preheat the oven to 125°F (50°C, or its lowest setting).

Spread the mixture very thinly on two baking sheets. Bake for about 6 hours, turning over halfway through to help the drying process. Remove from the oven and cool completely on the baking sheet.

Cut or break into pieces. The crackers can be stored in an airtight container for 2 to 4 weeks.

Variations

Seaweed and seed crackers: Follow the recipe as above, substituting 1 tbsp spirulina powder and 1 tbsp dried dulse flakes for the spice.

Curry and seed crackers: Follow the recipe above, substituting 1½ tbsp curry powder and 1 tsp garlic powder for the spice.

Sun-dried tomato and Italian herb crackers: Drain 12 sun-dried tomatoes packed in olive oil and pat dry. Process in a food processor until smooth. Follow the recipe above, substituting 1 tsp mixed Italian herbs, 1 tsp garlic powder, and the blended sun-dried tomatoes for the spice.

MACADAMIA CHEESE

MAKES 1 CUP (200 G)

1 heaping cup (155 g) macadamia nuts	2 tsp freshly squeezed lemon juice, plus more if needed

Soak the macadamia nuts in 3 cups (750 ml) water for at least 1 hour and up to 4 hours. Drain and rinse well.

Put the nuts in a food processor and add the lemon juice, ½ tsp sea salt, and a pinch of freshly cracked black pepper. Pulse for 1 minute to combine. Add ⅓ cup (80 ml) water and continue to process until smooth. Add more lemon juice if you prefer the cheese to be tangier. Transfer to a storage container and store in the fridge for 5 to 7 days.

CASHEW CHEESE

MAKES 1 CUP (200 G)

1 cup (155 g) cashews	2 tsp freshly squeezed lemon juice

Soak the cashews in 3 cups (750 ml) water for at least 1 hour and up to 4 hours. Drain and rinse well.

Put the nuts in a food processor and add the lemon juice, ½ tsp sea salt, and a pinch of freshly cracked black pepper. Pulse for 1 minute to combine. Add ¼ cup (60 ml) water and continue to process until smooth. Add more lemon juice if you prefer the cheese to be tangier. Transfer to a storage container and store in the fridge for 5 to 7 days.

MARINATED OLIVES

SERVES 2

1 tsp fennel seeds	Finely grated zest of 1 orange or lemon
1 tsp cumin seeds	
1 tsp coriander seeds	1 clove garlic, finely chopped
5 oz (115 g) mixed olives	Pinch of red chilli flakes, or to taste
⅔ cup (150 ml) good-quality extra virgin olive oil	Leaves from 1 to 2 sprigs rosemary
1 tbsp sherry vinegar	Several sprigs thyme

Combine the fennel, cumin, and coriander seeds in a dry frying pan and toast over medium heat, shaking the pan often to evenly distribute the spices, until fragrant, about 5 minutes.

In a bowl, combine the olives, oil, vinegar, orange zest, garlic, red chilli flakes, rosemary, thyme, ¼ tsp sea salt, and ¼ tsp freshly cracked black pepper. Add the toasted seeds and mix to combine. Marinate the olives for at least 1 hour or, for best results, overnight.

Store in a sterilized jar. If the olives are fully submerged in olive oil, they will keep for up to 1 month.

ROASTED RED PEPPERS

MAKES 2 ROASTED PEPPERS

2 red peppers

Preheat the oven to 450°F (230°C gas 8).

Place the peppers on a large baking sheet and roast for 20 to 30 minutes, or until the skins blister and turn slightly black. Remove from the oven, place in a bowl, and cover with plastic wrap. Or place the roasted peppers in a plastic bag until cool. Peel away the skins. Discard the core, seeds, and membrane. Use the roasted flesh as desired. Roasted peppers will keep in an airtight container in the refrigerator for up to 1 week.

CLEANING SQUID

1 whole squid

Remove the innards from the squid by pulling the tentacles from the body. Carefully remove the ink sac in one piece from innards and set aside for another use or discard. Cut across the head, underneath the eyes, to separate the tentacles in one piece (discard the innards and eyes). Push the tentacles outwards, squeeze the beak out, and discard. Slice off the wings from the body with a sharp knife and remove. Remove the skin on the body by running your finger underneath the skin, separating it from the flesh, then peeling it off in one piece and discarding. Remove the skin from the wings, trim the tough flesh, and set aside. Remove the backbone from the tube. Open the tube and scrape and discard the insides. Score halfway through the flesh with a sharp knife in a crosshatch pattern (take care not to cut all the way through) or as specified in the recipe.

ACTIVATING NUTS & SEEDS

MAKES 3¼ CUPS (500 G) ALMONDS, CASHEWS, HAZELNUTS, MACADAMIA NUTS, AND BRAZIL NUTS; 3 CUPS (500 G) PISTACHIO NUTS; AND 4 CUPS (500 G) SUNFLOWER SEEDS AND PUMPKIN SEEDS

1 lb (500 g) whole nuts
or seeds

Place the nuts in a bowl. Add enough filtered water to cover, then set aside to soak:

Almonds: 12 hours

Brazil nuts: 12 hours

Cashews: 2 to 4 hours

Hazelnuts: 12 hours

Macadamia nuts: 7 to 12 hours

Pecans: 4 to 6 hours

Pistachio nuts: 4 to 6 hours

Pumpkin seeds: 7 to 10 hours

Sunflower seeds: 2 hours

Walnuts: 4 to 8 hours

After soaking, the nuts or seeds will look nice and puffy and may even start to show signs of sprouting. Rinse the nuts or seeds under running water.

If you want to toast the nuts or seeds without damaging all those nutrients you've activated, you'll need to do so over low heat—either in a dehydrator or on the lowest temperature in your oven (at 120°F/50°C). This will take anywhere from 6 to 24 hours. The nuts or seeds are ready when they feel and taste dry.

Use your activated dried nuts or seeds as you normally would use toasted nuts or seeds. They last really well in an airtight container at room temperature. They can be ground, too.

LSA MEAL (RAW NUT & SEED MIX)

MAKES 8¼ CUPS (850 G)

3 cups (450 g) golden or brown linseeds

2 cups (250 g) sunflower seeds, activated

1 cup (155 g) almonds, activated

Place the linseeds, sunflower seeds, and almonds in a food processor and process on high for 2 to 3 minutes, or until fine crumbs form. Store in an airtight glass container in the fridge for up to 3 months.

SEGMENTING CITRUS

1 lime, lemon, orange, or other citrus fruit

Using a sharp paring knife, trim away the peel and pith without taking too much of the fruit. Cut against the membrane of the citrus flesh until you reach the centre of the fruit. Cut against the other side of the membrane and remove the segment with your knife. Do this with a bowl underneath to collect the juice and segments.

BACON BARK

MAKES 16 PIECES

8 rashers bacon, halved crosswise

⅓ cup (80 ml) maple syrup

3½ oz (100 g) raw cacao chocolate (page 210)

About ½ cup (60 g) pumpkin seeds, to sprinkle

Preheat the oven to 400° (200°C gas 6). Line a baking sheet with baking parchment.

Lay the bacon rashers in a single layer and brush with the maple syrup. Roast for 8 to 10 minutes, until crispy. Remove from the heat and allow to cool on the baking sheet.

While the bacon cools, in a heatproof bowl set over a saucepan filled with 1 inch (2.5 cm) of gently simmering water, melt the chocolate. Dip the bacon in the melted chocolate and place on a wire rack so excess chocolate can drip off. Sprinkle with pumpkin seeds and set aside to harden for a few minutes. Then serve or use as directed in a recipe.

SWEET PASTRY

MAKES ENOUGH FOR ONE 9-INCH (23 CM) PIE

½ cup (50 g) ground almonds
½ cup (50 g) coconut flour
¼ cup (30 g) arrowroot powder

10 tbsp (125 g) ghee or coconut oil, chilled and diced
3 tbsp raw honey
1 egg, lightly beaten

In a mixing bowl, combine the ground almonds, coconut flour, and arrowroot, and mix to combine. Using your hands, work the ghee into the dry ingredients to form fine crumbs. Add the honey and egg and mix to form a dough.

Transfer the dough to a work surface lightly dusted with arrowroot powder and knead the dough until it becomes nice and smooth (the dough may seem a little wet and sticky at first). Wrap in plastic wrap and refrigerate for 30 minutes, or until firm enough to roll out.

The pastry dough can be stored in a refrigerator for up to 1 week and in the freezer for 3 months.

Note: This recipe can also be used to make a savoury pastry. Just omit the honey and add a couple of pinches of sea salt and you have a savoury pastry that is perfect for savoury pies and quiches.

RAW CACAO CHOCOLATE

MAKES 1 LB (500 G)

1 cup (250 g) cocoa butter
1 cup (120 g) raw cacao powder, sifted

¼ cup plus 1 tbsp (90 g) raw honey

Line a baking sheet with baking parchment.

Put the cocoa butter in a heatproof bowl and set the bowl on top of a small saucepan filled with 2 inches (5 cm) of simmering water (make sure the water isn't touching the bowl) over medium heat. When the cocoa butter is completely melted, remove from the heat and add the cacao powder and honey. Mix until smooth. Make sure that no water or liquid gets into the chocolate, which would cause the texture to become grainy.

Pour the chocolate onto the prepared baking sheet and allow to sit for several hours at room temperature until set and hardened. You can also place it in the refrigerator to harden more quickly. Once hardened, remove it from the baking sheet, break it into pieces, and store in an airtight container for 2 or 3 weeks in the fridge.

CHOCOLATE SAUCE

MAKES 2½ CUPS (600 ML)

¾ cup plus 2 tbsp (300 g) raw honey
⅓ cup (80 ml) coconut oil

1 cup (120 g) raw cacao powder
⅔ cup (150 ml) coconut cream

Combine ½ cup (125 ml) warm water, the honey, and the coconut oil in a medium saucepan and bring to a boil over medium-high heat. Add the cacao and whisk until incorporated. Stir in the coconut cream. Strain through a fine-mesh sieve and allow to cool. Store in an airtight container in the fridge for up to 2 weeks.

WHIPPED COCONUT CREAM

MAKES 1¼ CUPS (230 G)

2 (15¼ oz/440 ml) cans coconut milk

2 tbsp raw honey, or to taste

Chill the coconut milk and a stainless steel stand mixer bowl in the refrigerator overnight. Open the cans and separate the cream layers from the water layer (reserve the water layer for another use). Combine the solidified cream layers and honey in the chilled bowl. Using a stand mixer fitted with the whisk attachment, whip the coconut cream on high speed until soft peaks form, 3 to 5 minutes. Allow to set in the fridge for 40 minutes before using.

PALEO VANILLA ICE CREAM

MAKES 1¼ QT (1.2 L)

1 tbsp gelatine powder
2 cups (500 ml) coconut cream
2 cups (500 ml) coconut milk

2 vanilla beans, split lengthwise and scraped
4 egg yolks
½ cup (170 g) raw honey or maple syrup

In a small bowl dissolve the gelatine in 3 tbsp of the coconut cream.

In a saucepan over medium-high heat, bring the remaining coconut cream, coconut milk, and vanilla bean to a boil, stirring occasionally. Stir in the gelatine mixture.

In a large bowl, whisk the egg yolks and honey together until fluffy and the colour lightens. While whisking constantly, pour half of the hot coconut mixture into the egg mixture. Whisk in the remaining hot coconut mixture and then pour the mixture back into another clean saucepan. Cook over medium heat, stirring with a wooden spoon or spatula, until the mixture thickens slightly and coats the back of the spoon, 5 to 8 minutes. Pour the mixture through a fine-mesh sieve into a bowl. Cover and refrigerate until very cold, at least 2 hours or up to overnight.

Pour the mixture into an ice cream maker and churn according to the manufacturer's directions. Transfer to an airtight container and freeze until firm. If the ice cream is too firm, put it in the refrigerator until it softens.

Variation

Chocolate ice cream: Follow the recipe as above, substituting ⅓ cup (40 g) raw cacao powder for the vanilla beans.

VANILLA MARSHMALLOWS

MAKES ABOUT 30 MARSHMALLOWS

Arrowroot powder or toasted unsweetened shredded dried coconut, to coat

3 tbsp plus ½ tsp unflavoured gelatine powder

1 cup (340 g) raw honey

1 egg white

½ tsp vanilla powder or 1 vanilla bean, split lengthwise and scraped

Line a 9 by 13-inch (23 by 33 cm) baking tin with baking parchment. Lightly dust the surface with arrowroot powder or toasted dried coconut.

In a small bowl, dissolve the gelatine in ½ cup (125 ml) water. Combine another ½ cup (125 ml) water and the honey in a saucepan over medium heat. Stir until the honey is dissolved. Continue to heat until the temperature reaches 250°F (121°C) on a sugar thermometer.

Meanwhile, in the bowl of a stand mixer fitted with the whisk attachment, beat the egg white at medium-high speed until it begins to fluff up. Add the gelatine mixture to the egg white with the machine running, then pour in the hot honey mixture gradually and in a steady stream. Beat in the vanilla powder or vanilla bean seeds. Continue to beat until soft peaks form and the mixture is velvety and bright white. Beat for about 5 minutes or until the mixture has cooled. Pour the marshmallow mixture into the prepared tin, and spread out evenly. Lightly dust more arrowroot over the top, transfer to the refrigerator, and let set for 2 hours. Cut into squares and serve.

ACKNOWLEDGEMENTS

This book is dedicated to everyone brave enough to step outside their comfort zone and embrace the Paleo way. Remember that 'food is medicine' or 'food is poison', and we all have the right to be healthy. It starts with a choice. Keep cooking for Life with Love and Laughter.

Thanks!

This book wouldn't have been possible without Nicola Robinson entering my life when she did. Thank you, Angel, for your love, support, wisdom, and belief in me to be the best I can be. I love you!

To my darling little 'bunnies', Chilli and Indii: You girls grow wiser and more beautiful every day and I look forward to seeing where your journey of life takes you . . . I am sure you will enrich so many lives.

To Hannah Rahill: Thank you for enabling me to create a book that I had in my mind exactly as I wanted it without dumbing it down or taking away the essence and message that I needed to express.

Mark Roper, you are a magician behind the lens! Thank you for the wonderful images that make the food jump off the page.

Deb Kaloper, the queen of styling, you definitely have a rare and special talent for making the food look so relaxed and accessible.

Kim Laidlaw, thank you for testing and correcting my words and recipes with your unwavering attention to detail.

To the wonder twins Monica & Jacinta: Once again you have evolved and grown as chefs and I am proud to have you both give up your time and help me out on this project.

Thank you to my mentors: Nora Gedgaudas, David Perlmutter, Rudolph Elkhardt, Pete Bablis, William Davis, Pete Melov, Bruce Fife, David Gillespie, Loren Cordain, Sandor Katz, Donna Gates, Sally Fallon, Weston A. Price, Mark Sisson, Robb Wolf, Joshua Rosenthal, Kitsa Yanniotis, and all the other passionate people who dedicate their lives to helping others.

And lastly to my mum, Joy: I love you!

INDEX

First published in the USA 2015 by Ten Speed Press,
an imprint of the Crown Publishing Group

First published in the UK 2015 by Macmillan
an imprint of Pan Macmillan
20 New Wharf Road, London N1 9RR
Associated companies throughout the world
www.panmacmillan.com

ISBN 978-1-4472-9833-5

A CIP catalogue record for this book is available from the British Library.

Design by Margaux Keres
Printed and bound in China